THE COMPLETE

MIND DIET

COOKBOOK

FOR BEGINNERS 2024

DELICIOUS AND TASTY RECIPES FOR BRAIN HEALTH AND WEIGHT MANAGEMENT

Marlene E. Martinez

THE COMPLETE
MIND DIET GUIDE

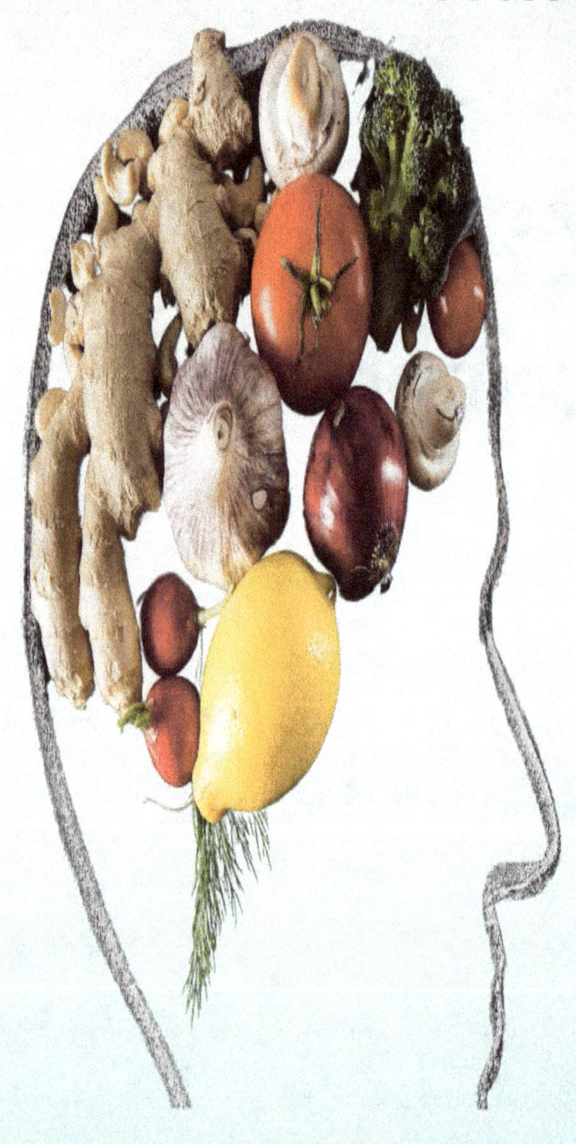

Copyright © Marlene E. Martinez 2024.

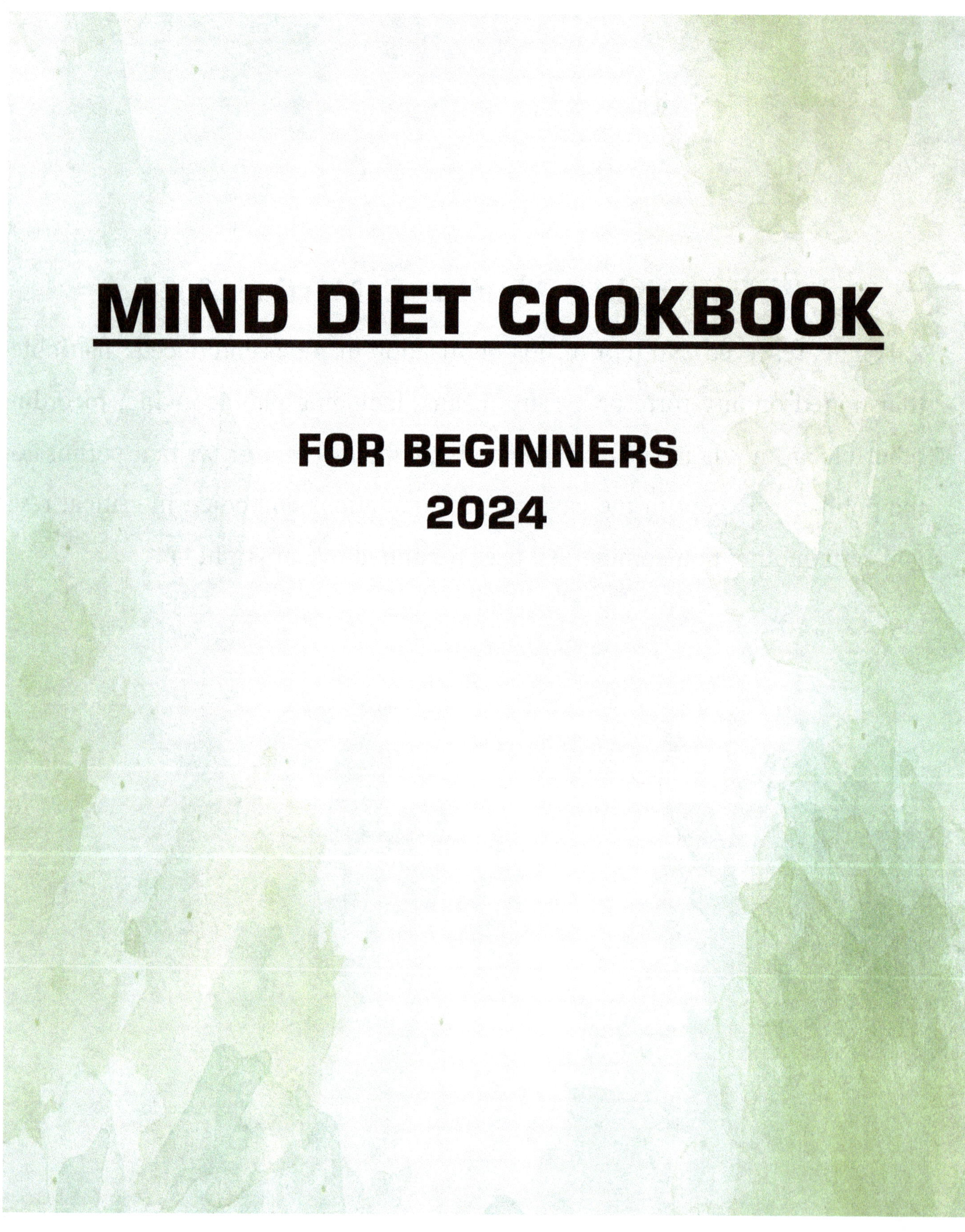

MIND DIET COOKBOOK

FOR BEGINNERS
2024

CONTENTS

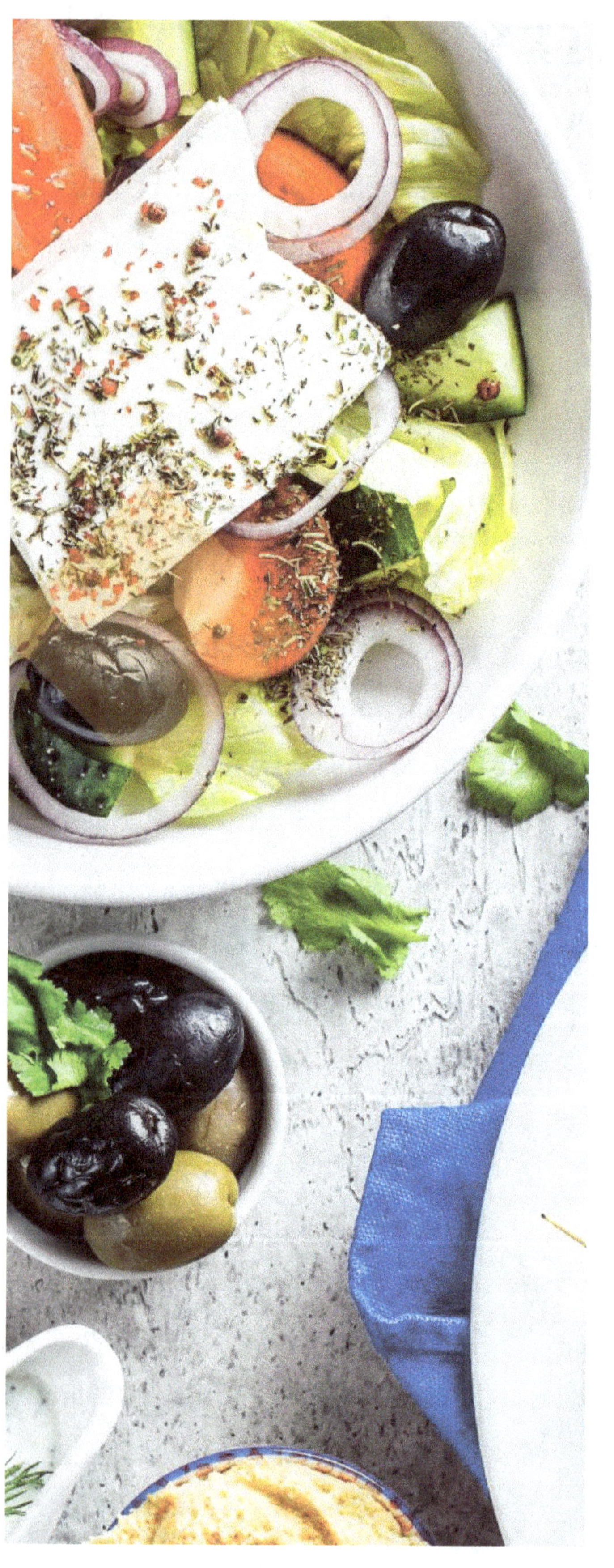

SECTION 1: INTRODUCTION

Understanding the Mind Diet

What is the Mind Diet?

The MIND Diet, which stands for "Mediterranean-DASH Intervention for Neurodegenerative Delay," is a dietary regimen that aims to improve brain health and lower the risk of cognitive decline and neurodegenerative disorders like Alzheimer's disease. It combines components of the Mediterranean Diet and the DASH (Dietary Approaches to Stop Hypertension) Diet, with a focus on specific foods linked to cognitive health.

The MIND Diet recommends eating green leafy vegetables, other vegetables, berries (especially blueberries and strawberries), nuts, whole grains, fish, poultry, olive oil, and alcohol in moderation. It also suggests minimizing your intake of red meat, butter and margarine, cheese, pastries and sweets, fried or fast food, and highly processed meals.

This dietary pattern is supported by studies that shows that the foods in the MIND Diet are high in nutrients and antioxidants, which may help protect the brain from oxidative stress, inflammation, and other processes related with cognitive decline. Following the MIND Diet may not only benefit brain function, but it may also improve overall well-being and lower the risk of chronic diseases.

Benefits of the Mind Diet for Brain Health

Reduced Risk of Alzheimer's Disease: According to several studies, following the MIND diet is connected with a lower risk of Alzheimer's disease and age-related cognitive decline. For example, a study published in Alzheimer's & Dementia discovered that people who closely followed the MIND diet had a slower pace of cognitive decline and a significantly reduced risk of getting Alzheimer's disease than those who followed the diet less rigorously.

Rich in Brain-Healthy Foods: The MIND diet focuses on foods that are especially favourable to brain health. These include leafy green vegetables, berries (particularly blueberries), almonds, whole grains, seafood, chicken, olive oil, and a moderate amount of wine. These meals are high in nutrients like antioxidants, omega-3 fatty acids, vitamins, and minerals, which have been found to improve cognitive performance and protect against neurodegeneration.

Anti-inflammatory Effects: The MIND diet, which emphasises whole, plant-based foods and healthy fats, is thought to help reduce inflammation throughout the body, including the brain. Chronic inflammation is becoming recognised as a risk factor for a variety of neurodegenerative disorders, including Alzheimer's. The MIND diet, by encouraging an anti-inflammatory environment, may help protect brain function and lower the risk of cognitive decline.

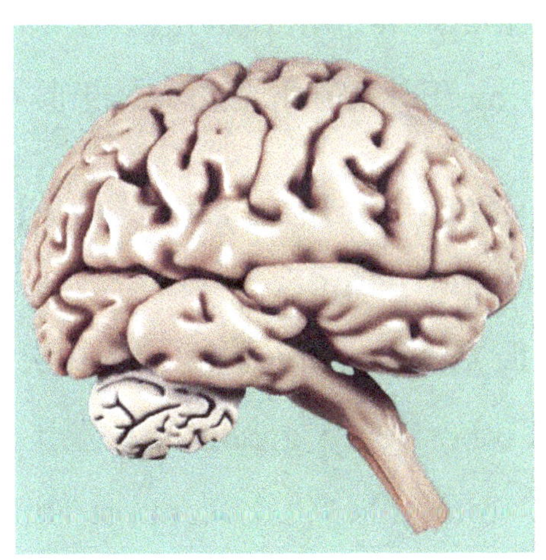

Heart Health Benefits: Similar to the Mediterranean and DASH diets, the MIND diet supports heart health. Many of the foods advised in the diet, such as fruits, vegetables, nuts, and fish, have been shown to benefit cardiovascular health by lowering blood pressure, cholesterol levels, and increasing blood vessel function. Because heart health is inextricably related to brain health, eating the MIND diet may indirectly boost cognitive performance by increasing overall cardiovascular function.

The MIND diet's adaptability and durability are two of its key characteristics. Unlike more restrictive diets, such as low-carb or ketogenic diets, the MIND diet allows for a wider range of foods and does not impose tight macronutrient ratios. This makes it easier for people to embrace and stick to in the long run, improving their chances of reaping the brain health benefits.

Foods to Include and Avoid

Foods to Include:

Leafy Greens: Spinach, kale, collard greens, and other leafy greens are rich in vitamins and minerals that support brain health, including folate, vitamin K, and antioxidants.

Berries: Blueberries, strawberries, raspberries, and blackberries are packed with antioxidants, particularly flavonoids, which

Promising Research Continues: While existing research on the MIND diet and brain health is promising, additional studies are being conducted to investigate its potential advantages and mechanisms of action. Researchers are examining how individual nutrients and dietary patterns affect brain function, as well as the role of the gut-brain axis in mediating these effects. Continued research in this area may provide more information about optimising dietary practices for maintaining cognitive function and lowering the risk of neurodegenerative disorders.

have been associated with improved cognitive function.

Nuts: Walnuts, almonds, pistachios, and other nuts are excellent sources of healthy fats, antioxidants, and vitamin E, all of which support brain health.

Fish: Fatty fish like salmon, trout, mackerel, and sardines are rich in omega-3 fatty acids, which are essential for brain function and may help reduce the risk of cognitive decline.

Whole Grains: Foods like whole wheat, oats, brown rice, and quinoa provide fiber, vitamins, and minerals that support overall health, including brain function.

Beans and Legumes: Lentils, chickpeas, black beans, and other legumes are high in fiber, protein, and nutrients that promote brain health.

Olive Oil: Extra virgin olive oil is a staple of the Mediterranean diet and is rich in monounsaturated fats and antioxidants, which are beneficial for brain health.

Poultry: Lean sources of poultry such as chicken and turkey are rich in protein and nutrients like vitamin B12, which may help protect against cognitive decline.

Wine (in moderation): Red wine, in moderation, has been associated with improved cognitive function due to its antioxidant properties, particularly resveratrol.

Herbs and Spices: Turmeric, cinnamon, oregano, and other herbs and spices contain antioxidants and anti-inflammatory compounds that may support brain health.

Foods to Avoid:

Red Meat: While not entirely off-limits, it's recommended to limit consumption of red meat and processed meats like bacon and sausage, as they are high in saturated fats and may increase the risk of cognitive decline.

Butter and Margarine: High intake of saturated and trans fats, found in butter and margarine, has been linked to an increased risk of Alzheimer's disease and other cognitive impairments.

Cheese: While cheese can be enjoyed in moderation, it's high in saturated fats and sodium, so it's best to limit consumption, especially of processed cheeses.

Sweets and Pastries: Foods high in added sugars and refined carbohydrates, such as cakes, cookies, candies, and pastries, should be limited as they may contribute to inflammation and cognitive decline.

Fried and Fast Foods: Fried foods like French fries, fried chicken, and fast food items are often high in unhealthy fats, sodium, and calories, which can have a negative impact on brain health over time.

Processed Foods: Foods high in additives, preservatives, and artificial ingredients, such as packaged snacks, frozen meals, and instant noodles, should be limited as they offer little nutritional value and may contribute to inflammation.

Excessive Salt: High intake of sodium, often found in processed and packaged foods, can lead to high blood pressure and may increase the risk of cognitive decline, so it's important to limit salt intake.

Sugary Beverages: Sodas, fruit juices with added sugars, energy drinks, and other sugary beverages should be avoided or consumed sparingly, as they offer little nutritional value and may contribute to cognitive decline.

Trans Fats: Foods containing partially hydrogenated oils, such as certain baked goods, fried foods, and processed snacks, should be avoided altogether, as they have been linked to inflammation and an increased risk of cognitive impairment.

Alcohol (in excess): While moderate consumption of alcohol, particularly red wine, has been associated with improved cognitive function, excessive alcohol intake can have detrimental effects on brain health, so it's important to drink in moderation.

SECTION 2: RECIPES

BREAKFAST BRAIN BOOSTERS

Blueberry Walnut Overnight Oats

Ingredients:

- 1 cup rolled oats (gluten-free if necessary)
- 1 cup unsweetened almond milk (or any milk of choice)
- 1/2 cup fresh blueberries
- 1/4 cup chopped walnuts
- 1 tablespoon chia seeds
- 1 tablespoon maple syrup (optional, depending on sweetness preference)
- 1/2 teaspoon vanilla extract
- Pinch of salt

Preparation Time: 10 minutes
Quantity: 2 servings

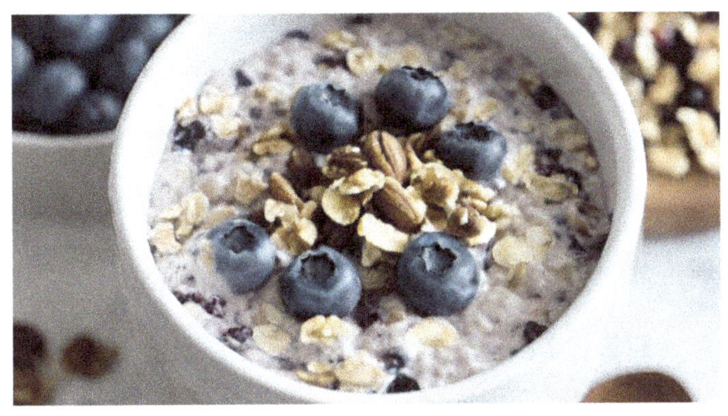

Instructions:

1. In a mixing dish or jar, mix together the rolled oats, almond milk, chia seeds, maple syrup (if using), vanilla essence, and a pinch of salt. Stir well to properly distribute all ingredients.

2. Gently stir in the fresh blueberries and chopped walnuts to the oat mixture.

3. Divide the mixture evenly between two airtight containers or jars.

4. Seal the containers firmly and chill overnight, or at least 4 hours, to allow the oats to soften and the flavours to combine.

5. Stir the overnight oats thoroughly in the morning before serving.

6. Before serving, you can add more fresh blueberries and chopped walnuts as garnish.

Spinach and Feta Egg Muffins

Ingredients:

- 6 large eggs
- 1 cup fresh spinach, chopped
- 1/2 cup crumbled feta cheese
- 1/4 cup diced red bell pepper
- 1/4 cup diced onion
- 1/4 teaspoon garlic powder
- Salt and pepper to taste
- Cooking spray or olive oil for greasing muffin tin

Prep Time: 10 minutes
Quantity: Makes 6 muffins

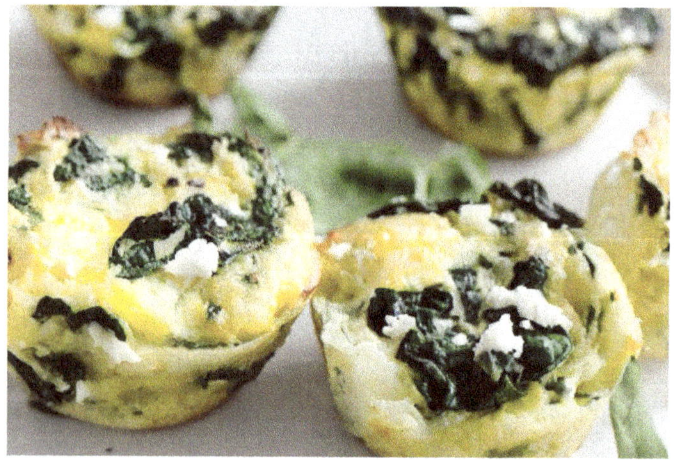

Instructions:

1. Preheat the oven to 350°F (175° C). Coat a muffin tray with cooking spray or olive oil.

2. In a mixing basin, crack the eggs and whisk until thoroughly blended.

3. Combine the chopped spinach, crumbled feta cheese, diced red bell pepper, diced onion, garlic powder, salt, and pepper with the eggs. Stir until the ingredients are uniformly distributed.

4. Pour the egg mixture equally into the prepared muffin cups, filling them about 3/4 full.

5. Place the muffin tin in the preheated oven for 20-25 minutes, or until the egg muffins are firm and faintly brown on top.

6. Once finished, remove the muffin tray from the oven and allow the egg muffins to cool for a few minutes.

7. Using a butter knife or spatula, slightly loosen the edges of the muffins before carefully removing them from the muffin tray.

8. Serve the spinach and feta egg muffins warm, or let them cool fully before

keeping in an airtight jar in the refrigerator for 3-4 days.

Avocado Toast with Smoked Salmon

Ingredients:

- 2 ripe avocados
- 4 slices of whole grain bread
- 100g smoked salmon
- 1 lemon
- 2 tablespoons chopped fresh dill
- Salt and pepper to taste

Preparation Time: 10 minutes

Quantity: Makes 4 servings

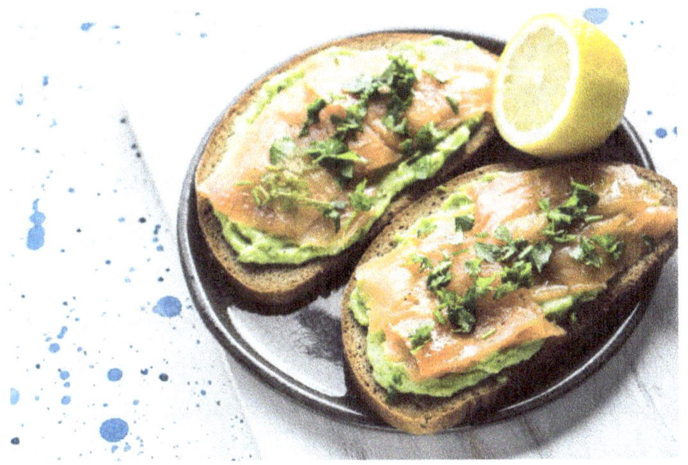

Instructions:

1. Begin by toasting the whole grain bread pieces to the desired crispiness. Set them aside once toasted.

2. Cut the avocados in half, take out the pits, and scoop the flesh into a basin. Mash the avocado with a fork until it's smooth but still somewhat lumpy.

3. Squeeze the juice of half a lemon into the mashed avocado and combine thoroughly. Season with salt and pepper to taste.

4. Spread the mashed avocado evenly on each slice of toasted bread.

5. Top each avocado toast with slices of smoked salmon, dividing them evenly.

6. Sprinkle chopped fresh dill over the smoked salmon.

7. If preferred, garnish with extra lemon slices to squeeze over the toast before serving.

8. Your mind is diet-friendly. Avocado Toast with Smoked Salmon is now ready to be enjoyed! Serve immediately for the greatest flavour and texture.

Greek Yogurt Parfait with Berries and Almonds

Ingredients:

- 1 cup Greek yogurt (preferably low-fat or non-fat)
- 1/2 cup mixed berries (such as strawberries, blueberries, raspberries)

- 2 tablespoons sliced almonds
- 1 tablespoon honey or maple syrup (optional, for added sweetness)
- 1/4 teaspoon vanilla extract (optional, for flavor enhancement)

Preparation Time: 5 minutes

Quantity: Makes 1 serving

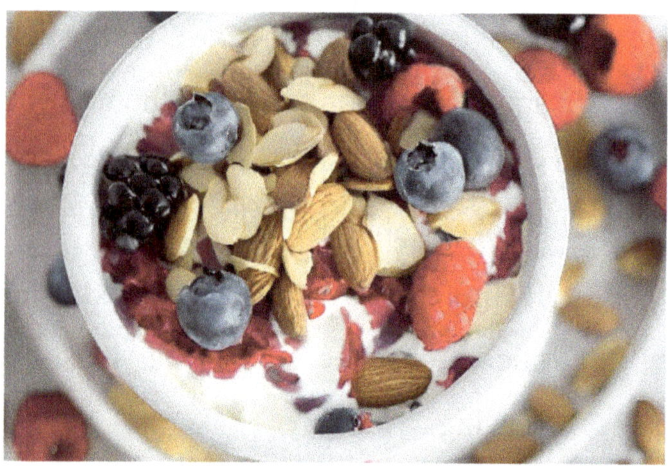

Instructions:

1. Prepare the Berries: Wash the berries in cold water and blot dry with a paper towel. If using strawberries, remove the stems and cut into smaller pieces if preferred.

2. Prepare the Yoghurt Mixture: In a mixing bowl, add Greek yoghurt, optional honey or maple syrup, and vanilla essence. Stir thoroughly to integrate. Adjust the sweetness to your liking.

3. Layering the Parfait: Grab a serving glass or bowl. Start by spooning a layer of Greek yoghurt mixture into the bottom of the glass.

4. Add the Berries: Spread a layer of mixed berries on top of the yoghurt. You can vary the varieties of berries for visual appeal.

5. Repeat Layers: Layer the Greek yoghurt mixture and berries till you reach the top of the glass, then top with a layer of yoghurt.

6. Garnish: Sprinkle sliced almonds on top of the parfait for a crisp texture and nutty flavour.

7. Serve: Your Greek Yoghurt Parfait with Berries and Almonds is ready to be enjoyed! Serve immediately as a healthy and enjoyable breakfast, snack, or dessert.

Quinoa Breakfast Bowl

Ingredients:

- 1 cup quinoa
- 2 cups of water or low-sodium vegetable broth
- 1 tablespoon olive oil
- 1 medium onion, diced
- 2 cloves garlic, minced
- 1 bell pepper, diced
- 1 cup spinach leaves, chopped
- 1 cup cherry tomatoes, halved
- 4 large eggs
- Salt and pepper to taste
- Optional toppings: sliced avocado, chopped fresh herbs (such as parsley or cilantro), feta cheese

Prep Time: 10 minutes

Quantity: Serves 4

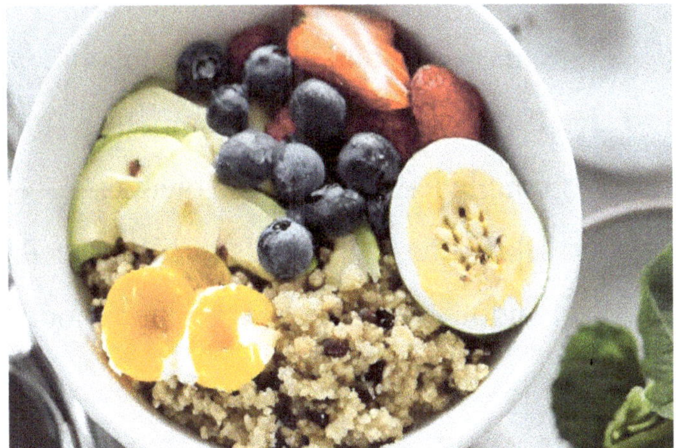

Instructions:

1. Rinse Quinoa: Place the quinoa in a fine-mesh strainer and rinse thoroughly with cold water.

2. To cook the quinoa, heat 2 cups of water or low-sodium vegetable broth in a medium saucepan until boiling. Add the rinsed quinoa, decrease the heat to low, cover, and simmer for 15-20 minutes, or until the quinoa is cooked and the liquid is absorbed. Remove from the heat and allow to settle for 5 minutes, covered. Fluff with a fork.

3. Sauté Vegetables: While the quinoa cooks, heat olive oil in a large skillet over medium heat. Cook until the onion is transparent, which should take around 3-4 minutes. Cook for an additional 1-2 minutes after adding the minced garlic. Cook for 2-3 minutes, until the diced bell pepper is slightly softened. Finally, add the chopped spinach and cherry tomatoes, cooking for another 2-3 minutes or until the spinach has wilted and the tomatoes

have softened. Season with salt and pepper to taste.

4. Cook eggs: In a separate nonstick skillet, cook or poach the eggs to your liking.

5. Assemble Bowls: Divide the cooked quinoa evenly between four bowls. Top each bowl with sautéed vegetables and a cooked egg. Add any desired toppings, such as sliced avocado, chopped fresh herbs, or crumbled feta cheese.

6. Serve the quinoa breakfast bowls immediately for a nutritious and delicious breakfast.

Green Smoothie

Ingredients:

- 2 cups fresh spinach leaves
- 1 ripe banana, peeled
- 1/2 avocado, peeled and pitted
- 1/2 cup fresh or frozen pineapple chunks
- 1 tablespoon chia seeds
- 1 cup unsweetened almond milk or coconut water
- Ice cubes (optional, for a colder smoothie)

Prep Time: 5 minutes
Quantity: Makes 2 servings

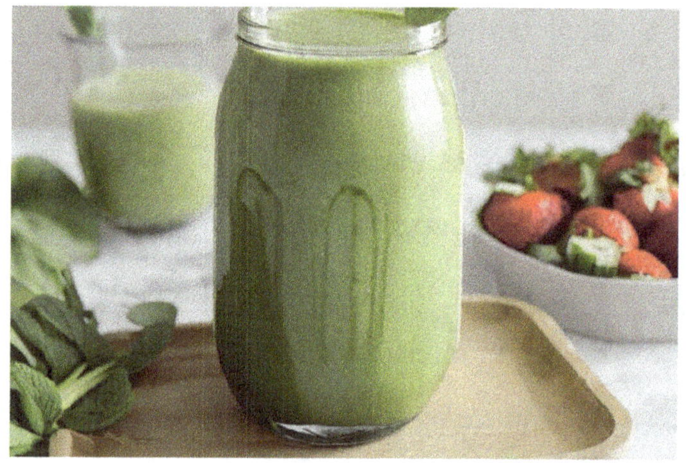

Instructions:

1. Wash the spinach leaves well in cold water and blot dry with paper towels.

2. In a blender, combine the spinach leaves, ripe banana, avocado, pineapple pieces, chia seeds, and almond or coconut water.

3. If you like a cooler smoothie, place a couple ice cubes in the blender.

4. Blend the ingredients at high speed until smooth and creamy. If the smoothie is too thick, add more almond milk or coconut water until you get the appropriate consistency.

5. Once combined, taste the smoothie and adjust the sweetness by adding extra banana or pineapple as needed.

6. Pour green smoothie into glasses and serve immediately. Enjoy your nutritious and delicious green smoothie as part of your Mind Diet regimen!

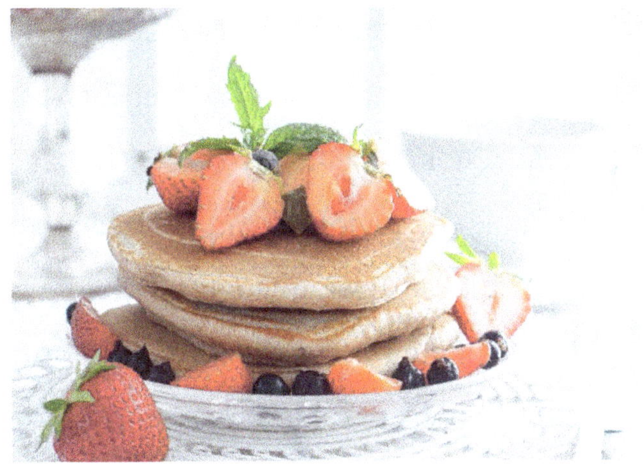

Whole Grain Pancakes with Mixed Berries

Ingredients:

- 1 cup whole grain pancake mix
- 1 cup mixed berries (such as strawberries, blueberries, raspberries)
- 1 tablespoon honey or maple syrup (optional)
- 1 cup low-fat or non-fat milk
- 1 large egg
- 1 tablespoon vegetable oil or melted butter
- Cooking spray or additional oil for greasing the pan

Prep Time: 15 minutes
Quantity: Makes about 8 pancakes

Instructions:

1. Prepare berries: Rinse the mixed berries in cold water and blot dry with a paper towel.

2. Preheat the griddle or pan: Preheat a nonstick griddle or skillet to medium heat. If using a skillet, coat it with cooking spray or a small amount of oil to prevent sticking.

3. Prepare the pancake batter: In a mixing bowl, combine the whole grain pancake mix, milk, egg, and vegetable oil/melted butter. Stir just until mixed. Be careful not to overmix; a few lumps are fine.

4. Cook Pancakes: When the griddle or skillet is hot, spoon 1/4 cup batter onto the cooking surface for each pancake. Cook the pancakes until bubbles appear on the surface, then turn them with a spatula and cook until golden brown on the opposite side. This usually takes around 2-3 minutes per side.

5. Serve: Stack the cooked pancakes onto a dish. Top the pancakes with the mixed berries. Drizzle with honey or maple syrup as desired.

6. Serve immediately and enjoy!

Chia Seed Pudding with Mango

Ingredients:

- 1/4 cup chia seeds
- 1 cup unsweetened almond milk (or any milk of your choice)
- 1 ripe mango, diced
- 1 tablespoon honey or maple syrup (optional, adjust according to taste)
- 1/2 teaspoon vanilla extract (optional)

Prep Time: 5 minutes

Quantity: 2 servings

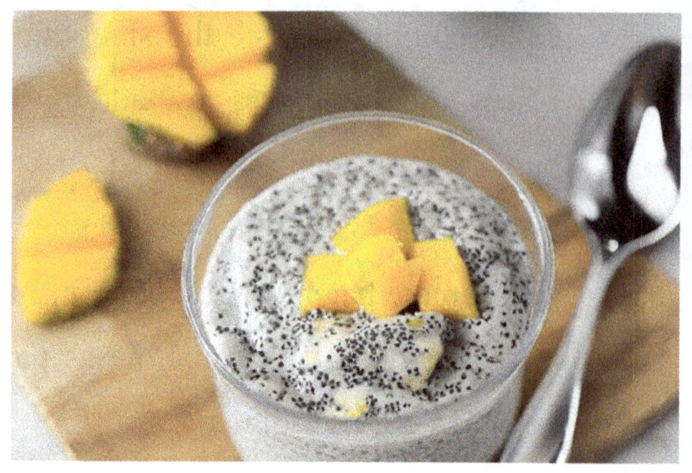

Instructions:

1. In a mixing bowl, combine the chia seeds and almond milk. Stir thoroughly to mix. For added sweetness and flavour, add honey or maple syrup, as well as vanilla essence. Mix thoroughly.

2. Allow the mixture to sit for approximately 5 minutes before stirring again to prevent clumping. Repeat this process a few more times over the next 15-20 minutes to ensure that the chia seeds absorb the liquid evenly.

3. Cover the bowl and chill for at least 2 hours, preferably overnight, to allow the pudding to thicken and set.

4. Once the chia pudding has set, whisk it thoroughly to release it. Taste and adjust the sweetness if necessary.

5. To serve, divide the chia seed pudding into serving bowls or glasses. Top each serving with diced mango.

6. Enjoy your nutritious and tasty chia seed pudding with mango as a delightful snack or breakfast choice that is suited for individuals on the Mind Diet.

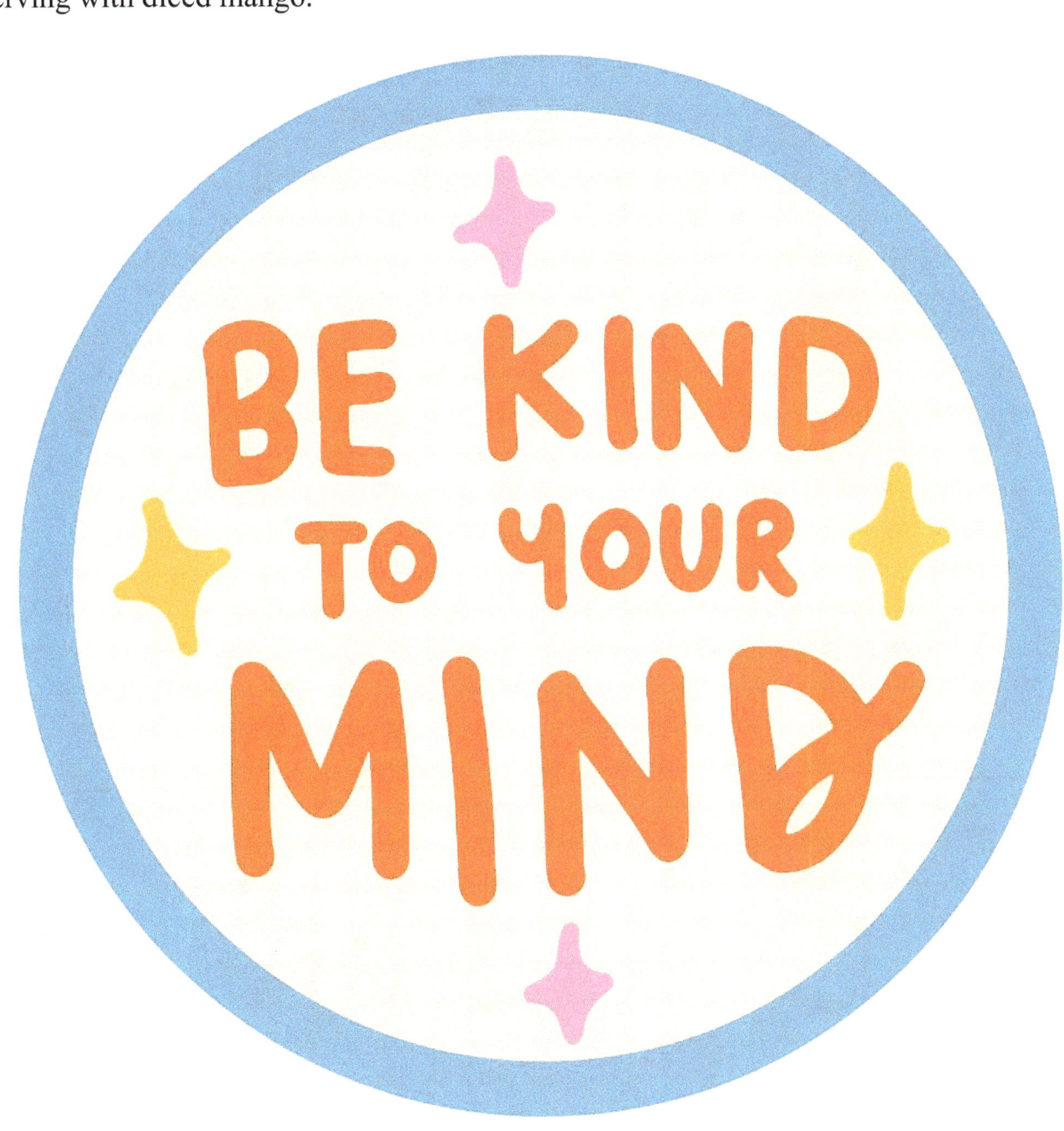

WHOLESOME LUNCH IDEAS

Salmon Salad:

Ingredients:

- 2 wild-caught salmon fillets (about 6 ounces each)
- 4 cups mixed salad greens (spinach, kale, arugula, etc.)
- 1 cup cherry tomatoes, halved
- 1 cucumber, sliced
- 1/4 cup red onion, thinly sliced
- 1/4 cup toasted walnuts, chopped
- 2 tablespoons fresh dill, chopped
- 2 tablespoons extra virgin olive oil
- 1 tablespoon lemon juice
- Salt and pepper to taste

Prep Time: 20 minutes
Quantity: Serves 2

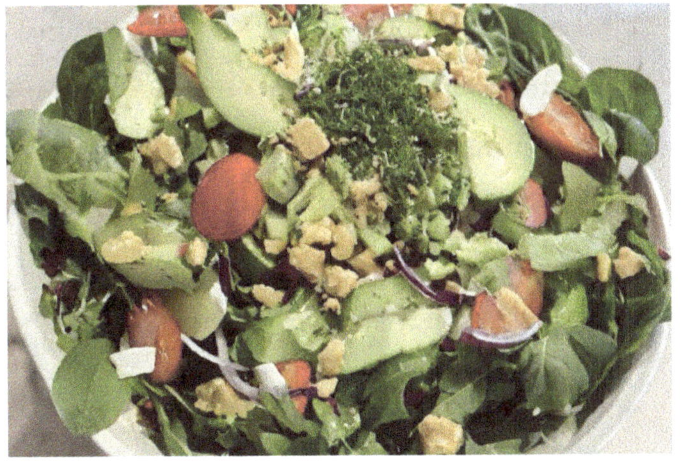

Instructions:

1. Preheat the oven to 375°F (190° C). Line a baking sheet with parchment paper.
2. Place the salmon fillets on the prepared baking sheet, skin side down. Season with salt and pepper.
3. Bake the salmon in a preheated oven for 12-15 minutes, or until well cooked and flaky. Once done, remove from the oven and allow it cool slightly.
4. While the salmon bakes, prepare the salad ingredients. In a large mixing bowl, add the mixed salad greens, cherry tomatoes, cucumber slices, red onion slices, toasted walnuts, and fresh dill.
5. The dressing is made by whisking together extra virgin olive oil and lemon juice in a small bowl. Season with salt and pepper to taste.
6. Once the salmon has cooled sufficiently, use a fork to break it up into bite-sized pieces.
7. Add the flakes salmon to the salad bowl.
8. Drizzle the dressing over the salad and gently toss to coat everything evenly.

9. Divide the salmon salad across two dishes and serve immediately.

Quinoa and Vegetable Stir-Fry:

Ingredients:

- 1 cup quinoa
- 2 cups water
- 2 tablespoons olive oil
- 2 cloves garlic, minced
- 1 onion, thinly sliced
- 1 bell pepper, thinly sliced
- 2 carrots, thinly sliced
- 1 zucchini, thinly sliced
- 1 cup broccoli florets
- 1 cup snap peas
- 1 tablespoon low-sodium soy sauce
- 1 tablespoon rice vinegar
- 1 teaspoon sesame oil
- Salt and pepper to taste
- Fresh cilantro or parsley for garnish (optional)

Preparation Time: 10 minutes
Quantity: Serves 4

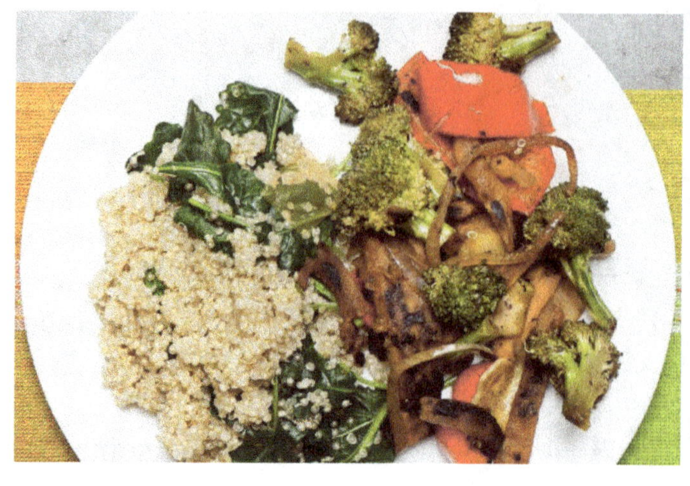

Instructions:

1. Prepare Quinoa: Rinse the quinoa in cold water through a fine mesh strainer. In a saucepan, mix the quinoa and water. Bring to a boil. Reduce the heat to low, cover, and cook for approximately 15 minutes, or until the water has been absorbed and the quinoa is fluffy. Remove from heat and cover for 5 minutes. Fluff with a fork.

2. Prepare stir-fry: Heat the olive oil in a large skillet or wok over medium-high heat. Combine the minced garlic and cut onion. Sauté for 2-3 minutes, until fragrant and the onions are transparent. Add the sliced bell pepper, carrots, zucchini, broccoli florets, and snap peas

to the skillet. Stir-fry the vegetables for 5-7 minutes, or until soft and crisp.

3. Combine: Add the cooked quinoa to the skillet along with the vegetables. Pour the low-sodium soy sauce, rice vinegar, and sesame oil over the mixture. Season with salt and pepper to taste. Toss everything together until thoroughly blended and cooked, about 2-3 minutes.

4. Serve: Transfer the quinoa and veggie stir-fry to individual serving dishes. Garnish with fresh cilantro or parsley if preferred.

Turkey and Avocado Wrap

Ingredients:

- 4 large whole wheat or spinach tortillas
- 2 ripe avocados, sliced
- 1 pound (about 450g) sliced turkey breast
- 1 cup shredded lettuce
- 1/2 cup diced tomatoes
- 1/4 cup thinly sliced red onion
- 1/4 cup chopped fresh cilantro (optional)
- 1/4 cup low-fat Greek yogurt or hummus
- Salt and pepper to taste

Prep Time: 15 minutes

Quantity: Makes 4 wraps

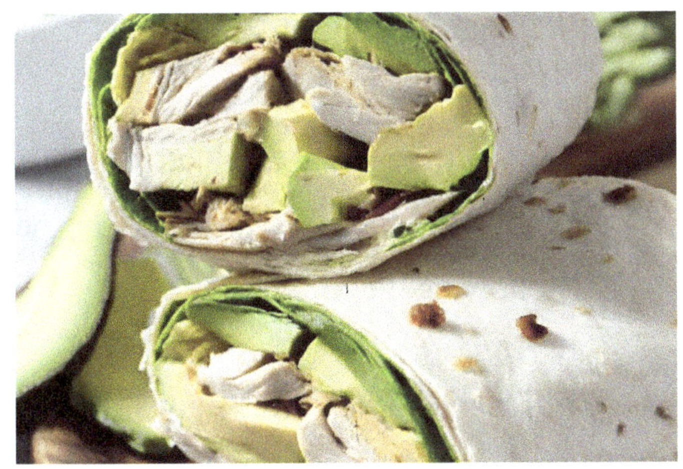

Instructions:

1. Arrange the tortillas on a clean surface. Spread a spoonful of Greek yoghurt or hummus evenly on each tortilla, leaving an inch boundary around the borders.

2. Divide the sliced avocado, turkey breast, shredded lettuce, chopped tomatoes, red onion, and cilantro (if using) evenly among the tortillas.

3. Season with salt and pepper to taste. Starting at one end, tightly roll up each tortilla, tucking in the sides as you go, to make a wrap.

4. Cut each wrap in half diagonally and serve right once, or wrap tightly in plastic wrap or foil for later use.

5. Enjoy these tasty and nutritious Turkey and Avocado Wraps, ideal for people following the Mind Diet!

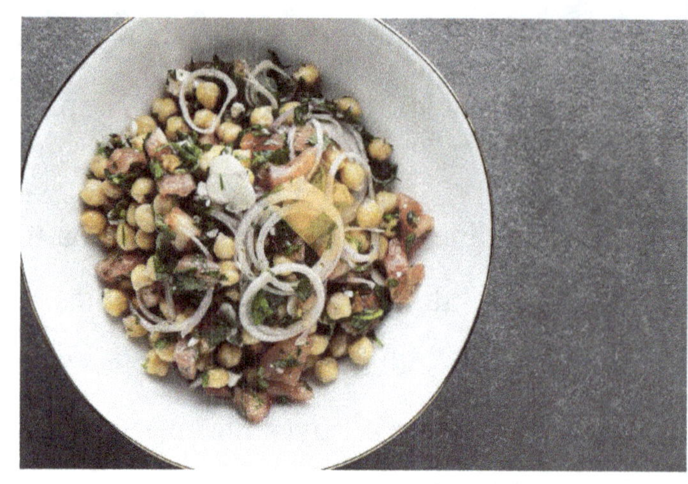

Mediterranean Chickpea Salad

Ingredients:

- 2 cans (15 oz each) chickpeas, drained and rinsed
- 1 cup cherry tomatoes, halved
- 1 cucumber, diced
- 1/2 red onion, thinly sliced
- 1/4 cup Kalamata olives, pitted and sliced
- 1/4 cup fresh parsley, chopped
- 1/4 cup fresh mint leaves, chopped
- 1/2 cup crumbled feta cheese (optional)
- 1/4 cup extra virgin olive oil
- 2 tablespoons red wine vinegar
- 1 clove garlic, minced
- Salt and black pepper to taste

Preparation Time: 15 minutes

Quantity: Serves 4

Instructions:

1. In a large mixing basin, mix together the chickpeas, cherry tomatoes, cucumber, red onion, Kalamata olives, parsley, and mint leaves.

2. If using, sprinkle crumbled feta cheese over the salad components.

3. To prepare the dressing, mix together the extra virgin olive oil, red wine vinegar, minced garlic, salt, and black pepper in a small bowl.

4. Pour the dressing over the salad and gently toss until everything is uniformly coated.

5. Taste and adjust seasoning as needed.

6. Serve immediately as a refreshing salad, or chill in the refrigerator for 30 minutes to allow the flavours to combine before serving.

Spinach and Mushroom Omelette

Ingredients:

- 2 large eggs
- 1 cup fresh spinach, chopped
- 1/2 cup mushrooms, sliced
- 1/4 cup onion, finely chopped
- 1 garlic clove, minced
- 1 tablespoon olive oil
- Salt and pepper to taste
- 1/4 cup shredded low-fat cheese (optional)

Preparation Time: 10 minutes

Cooking Time: 10 minutes

Quantity: 1 serving

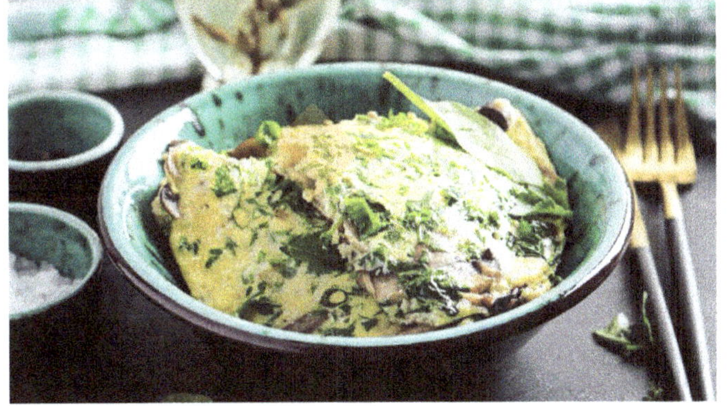

Instructions:

1. Prepare Ingredients:

Wash the spinach thoroughly before chopping it finely.

Slice the mushrooms, and finely chop the onion and garlic.

2. Sauté vegetables.

In a nonstick skillet, heat olive oil over medium heat.

Add the chopped onions and minced garlic to the skillet. Sauté until fragrant and the onions are transparent, about 2-3 minutes.

Cook the sliced mushrooms until they begin to brown, about 3-4 minutes.

3. Add spinach:

After the mushrooms have browned slightly, add the chopped spinach to the skillet.

Cook for about 2-3 minutes, or until the spinach is wilted and any excess liquid has evaporated.

Season with salt and pepper to taste.

4. Prepare eggs:

In a mixing dish, combine the eggs and beat well.

Pour the beaten eggs onto the sautéed vegetables in the skillet.

5. Cook an omelette:

Allow the eggs to set somewhat around the edges before carefully lifting them with a spatula to let the uncooked eggs flow below. Continue to cook until the omelette is mostly set but still somewhat runny on top.

6. Fold and serve.

Using a spatula, carefully fold the omelette in half.

Transfer the omelette to a platter and serve hot.

Tuna and White Bean Salad:

Ingredients:

- 2 cans (5 ounces each) of water-packed tuna, drained
- 2 cans (15 ounces each) of white beans (such as cannellini or navy beans), drained and rinsed
- 1 cup cherry tomatoes, halved
- 1/2 red onion, thinly sliced
- 2 tablespoons chopped fresh parsley
- 2 tablespoons extra-virgin olive oil
- 2 tablespoons lemon juice
- 1 clove garlic, minced
- Salt and pepper to taste
- Optional: 1/4 cup chopped olives or capers for extra flavor
- Optional: Mixed salad greens for serving

Preparation Time: 15 minutes
Quantity: 4 servings

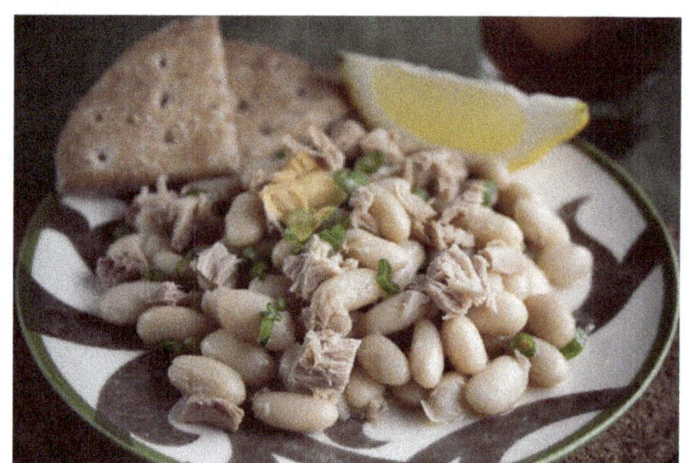

Instructions:

1. In a large mixing bowl, combine drained tuna, white beans, cherry tomatoes, sliced red onion, and parsley. If using, include the chopped olives or capers.

2. Whisk together the extra-virgin olive oil, lemon juice, minced garlic, salt, and pepper to make the dressing.

3. Pour the dressing over the tuna-white bean mixture. Gently toss until all ingredients are well coated in the dressing.

4. Taste and adjust seasoning as needed.

5. If desired, serve the tuna and white bean salad over a bed of mixed salad greens, or eat it as is.

6. Refrigerate any leftovers in an airtight jar for up to two days.

Sweet Potato and Black Bean Quesadillas:

Ingredients:

- 2 medium sweet potatoes, peeled and diced

- 1 can (15 ounces) black beans, rinsed and drained

- 1 red bell pepper, diced

- 1 small red onion, diced

- 2 cloves garlic, minced

- 1 teaspoon ground cumin

- 1 teaspoon chili powder

- Salt and pepper, to taste

- 4 whole grain or whole wheat tortillas

- 1 cup shredded reduced-fat cheese (such as cheddar or Mexican blend)

- Cooking spray or olive oil for cooking

Prep Time: 20 minutes

Quantity: Makes 4 quesadillas

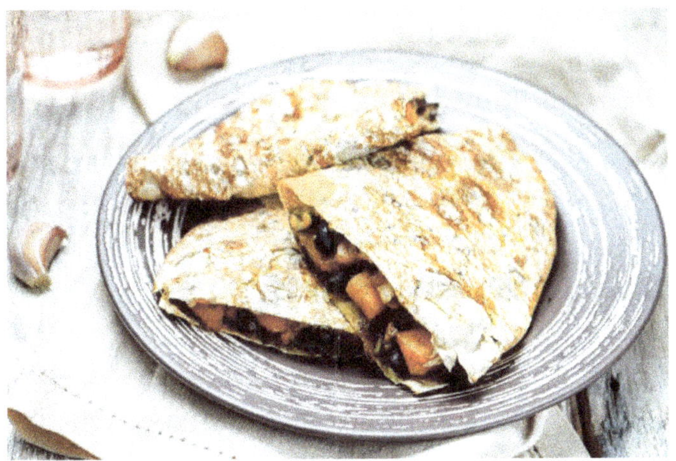

Instructions:

1. Prepare sweet potatoes: In a medium saucepan, cook diced sweet potatoes until cooked, about 10-15 minutes. Drain and set aside.

2. Cook the onion and bell pepper in a large skillet over medium heat, using a small amount of olive oil or cooking spray. Cook for 5 minutes, or until the diced red onion and red bell pepper soften. Cook for one more minute after adding the minced garlic.

3. Combine the cooked sweet potatoes, black beans, ground cumin, chilli powder, salt, and pepper in the skillet with the onion and bell pepper. Stir well to mix, then simmer for an additional 2-3 minutes until thoroughly cooked. Mash some of the sweet potatoes and beans with a fork to get a slightly lumpy mixture.

4. To assemble quesadillas, place one tortilla on a flat surface. Spread a quarter of the sweet potato and black bean mixture evenly on one half of the tortilla. Sprinkle with one-quarter of the shredded cheese. Fold the empty side of the tortilla over the filling to form a half moon shape.

5. Cook Quesadillas: Wipe out the skillet used for the filling, or use a new large skillet. Spray with cooking spray or drizzle with olive oil and place over medium heat. Cook one formed quesadilla in a skillet until golden brown and crispy on one side, about 2-3 minutes. Flip carefully and cook the second side for another 2-3 minutes, or until golden brown and the cheese has melted. Repeat for the remaining quesadillas.

6. Serve: Once done, remove the quesadillas from the skillet and let cool slightly before cutting into wedges. Serve warm, with salsa, guacamole, or Greek yoghurt to dip.

Greek Yogurt Chicken Salad:

Ingredients:

- 2 cups cooked chicken breast, shredded or diced
- 1 cup Greek yogurt (low-fat or non-fat)
- 1/4 cup diced red onion
- 1/4 cup diced cucumber
- 1/4 cup diced bell pepper (any color)
- 1/4 cup diced celery
- 1/4 cup chopped fresh parsley
- 1/4 cup chopped walnuts
- 1 tablespoon lemon juice
- 1 teaspoon Dijon mustard
- Salt and pepper to taste
- Optional: 1/4 cup diced apple or grapes for sweetness

Preparation Time: 15 minutes

Quantity: This recipe makes about 4 servings.

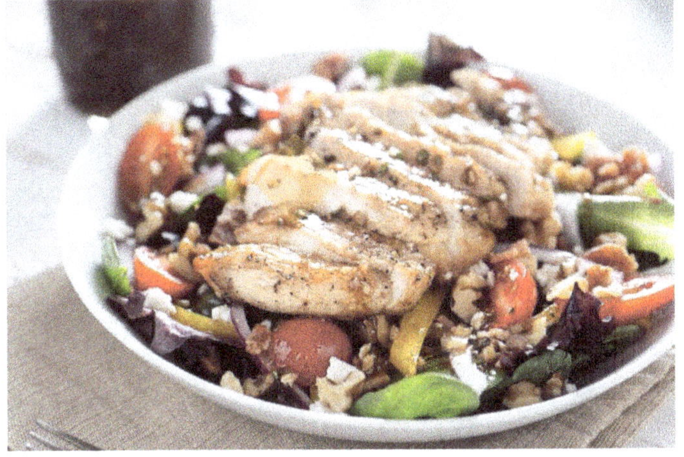

Instructions:

1. In a large mixing basin, mix together the Greek yoghurt, lemon juice, Dijon mustard, salt, and pepper. Stir until thoroughly blended.

2. Add the cooked chicken breast to the bowl and stir until evenly covered with the yoghurt mixture.

3. In the bowl, combine the diced red onion, cucumber, bell pepper, celery, chopped parsley, chopped walnuts, and any optional diced apples or grapes. Mix until all components are thoroughly blended.

4. Taste the chicken salad and, if necessary, season with extra salt, pepper, or lemon juice.

5. Once seasoned to your desire, wrap the bowl with plastic wrap or transfer the chicken salad to an airtight container. Refrigerate for at least 30 minutes before serving to let the flavours to combine.

6. Serve chilled as a sandwich filler, over a bed of greens, or with whole grain crackers.

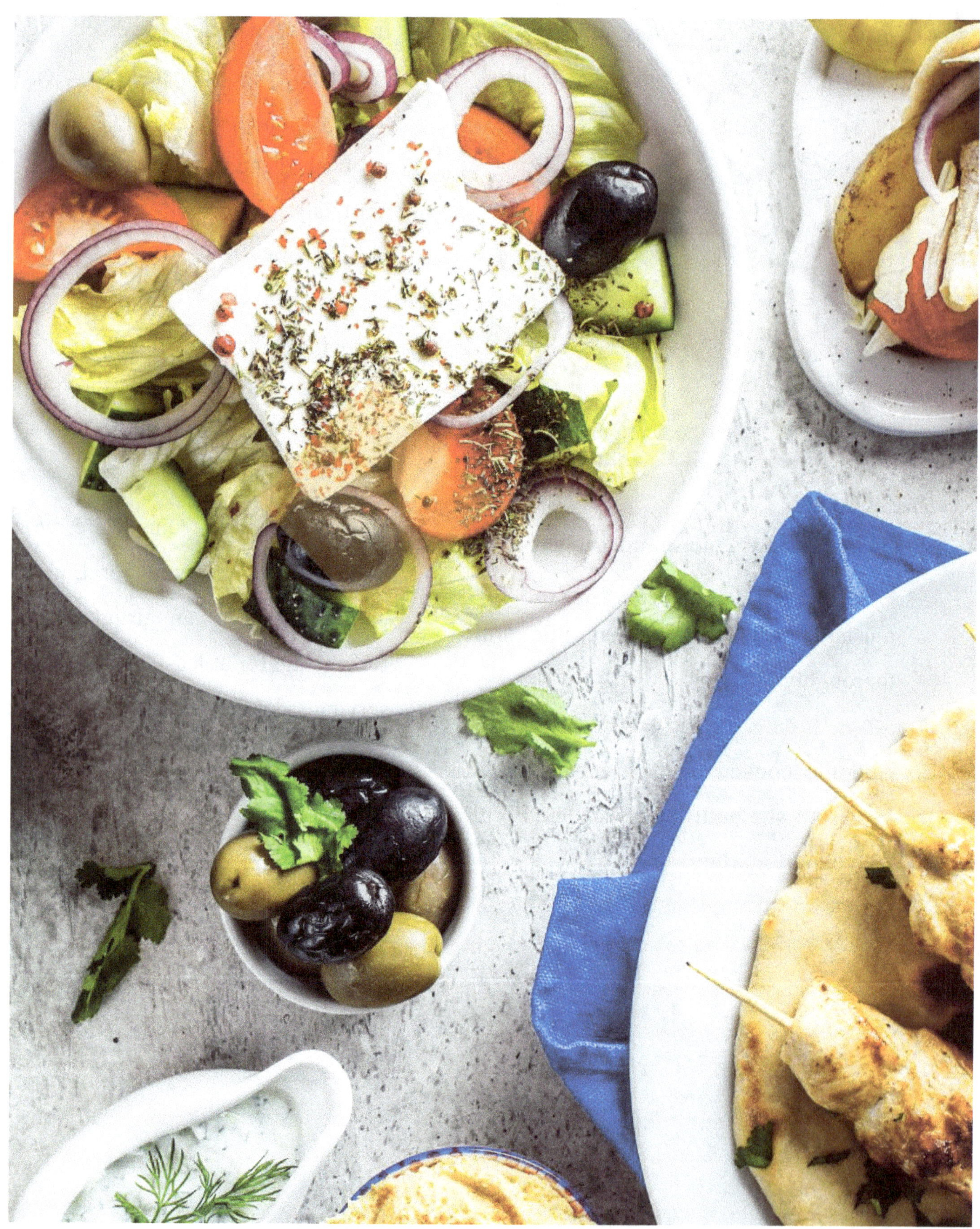

NOURISHING DINNER RECIPES

Lentil and Vegetable Curry

Ingredients:

- 1 cup dry green or brown lentils, rinsed
- 2 cups vegetable broth (low sodium)
- 1 tablespoon olive oil
- 1 onion, diced
- 3 cloves garlic, minced
- 1 tablespoon grated fresh ginger
- 2 carrots, diced
- 2 stalks celery, diced
- 1 bell pepper, diced
- 1 zucchini, diced
- 1 can (14 oz) diced tomatoes (no salt added)
- 2 tablespoons tomato paste
- 2 teaspoons ground cumin
- 1 teaspoon ground coriander
- 1 teaspoon turmeric
- 1 teaspoon paprika
- 1/2 teaspoon cinnamon
- Salt and pepper to taste
- Fresh cilantro leaves for garnish (optional)

Preparation Time: 10 minutes

Cooking Time: 35 minutes

Quantity: Serves 4

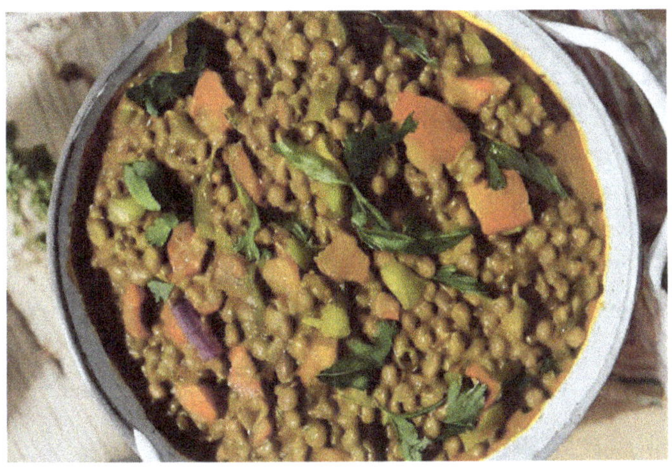

Instructions:

1. Prepare the lentils: In a medium saucepan, combine the rinsed lentils with the vegetable broth. Bring to a boil over medium high heat. Reduce the heat to low, cover, and cook for 20-25 minutes, until the lentils are cooked but not mushy. Drain the extra liquid and set it aside.

2. Sauté Aromatics: Warm olive oil in a large skillet or pot over medium heat. Sauté the diced onion until transparent, about 3-4 minutes. Add the minced

garlic and grated ginger and simmer for another minute until fragrant.

3. Stir in the diced carrots, celery, bell pepper, and zucchini. Cook for 5-7 minutes until the vegetables soften.

4. Spice It Up: Add diced tomatoes, juices, and tomato paste to the skillet. Stir in the ground cumin, coriander, turmeric, paprika, cinnamon, salt, and pepper. Mix thoroughly to mix.

5. Simmer: Bring the mixture to a simmer, then turn the heat down to low. Cover and boil slowly for 10-15 minutes, allowing the flavours to mingle and the veggies to soften.

6. Combine Lentils and Vegetables: Once the vegetables have reached your desired softness, add the cooked lentils to the skillet. Stir thoroughly to combine all of the ingredients.

7. Adjust seasoning: Taste the curry and, if necessary, add additional salt or spices to your liking.

8. Serve by removing from the heat. Garnish with fresh cilantro leaves if desired. Serve hot with cooked brown rice or quinoa, or on its own as a substantial stew.

Stuffed Bell Peppers with Ground Turkey and Brown Rice

Ingredients:

- 4 large bell peppers, any color
- 1 pound ground turkey
- 1 cup cooked brown rice
- 1 small onion, finely chopped
- 2 cloves garlic, minced
- 1 cup diced tomatoes (fresh or canned)
- 1/2 cup low-sodium chicken or vegetable broth
- 1 teaspoon dried oregano
- 1 teaspoon dried basil
- Salt and pepper to taste
- Optional: 1/2 cup shredded low-fat mozzarella cheese
- Fresh parsley for garnish (optional)

Prep Time: 20 minutes

Cook: 40 minutes

Total: 1 hour

Quantity: Serves: 4

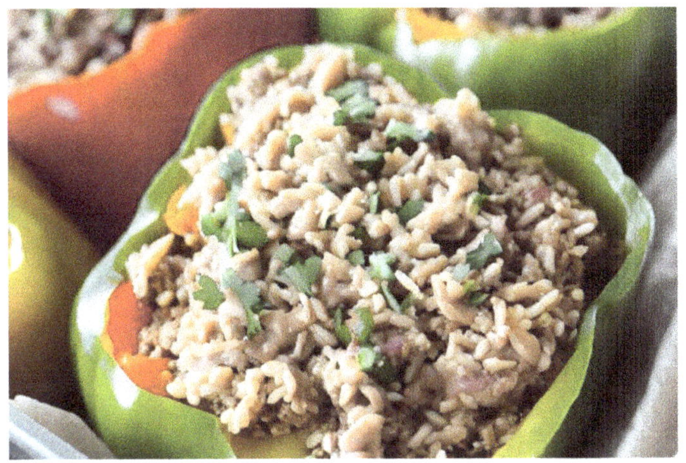

Instructions:

1. Preheat the oven. Preheat the oven to 375°F (190° C).

2. Prepare the bell peppers by cutting off the tops and removing the seeds and membranes. Rinse the peppers with cool water and set aside.

3. Prepare the Filling: Cook the ground turkey in a skillet over medium heat until no longer pink, breaking it up with a spoon as it cooks. Drain any extra fat as needed.

4. Cook Aromatics: In the same skillet, combine the chopped onion and minced garlic. Sauté until softened, about 3-4 minutes.

5. Combine the ingredients and return the cooked turkey to the skillet. Combine the cooked brown rice, diced tomatoes, dried oregano, dry basil, salt, and pepper. Stir thoroughly to mix.

6. Fill the Bell Peppers: Arrange the bell peppers upright in a baking dish. Spoon the turkey and rice mixture into each pepper, filling them completely.

7. Add Liquid: Pour the chicken or vegetable broth into the baking dish, surrounding the peppers. This helps keep the peppers moist as they bake.

8. Cover the baking dish with aluminium foil and bake in a preheated oven for 30-35 minutes, or until the peppers are soft.

9. Optional Cheese Topping: Remove the foil during the last 5 minutes of baking

and sprinkle shredded mozzarella cheese on top of the peppers. Return to the oven until the cheese has melted and bubbled.

10. Serve: Once cooked, take the peppers from the oven and allow to cool slightly before serving. Garnish with fresh parsley if preferred.

Salmon with Quinoa and Steamed Vegetables

Ingredients:

- 4 salmon fillets (about 6 ounces each), skinless
- 1 cup quinoa, rinsed
- 2 cups mixed vegetables (such as broccoli, carrots, and bell peppers), chopped
- 2 tablespoons olive oil
- 2 cloves garlic, minced
- 1 lemon, juiced
- Salt and pepper to taste
- 1 teaspoon dried herbs (such as thyme or rosemary), optional
- Lemon wedges, for serving

Prep Time: 15 minutes

Quantity: Serves 4

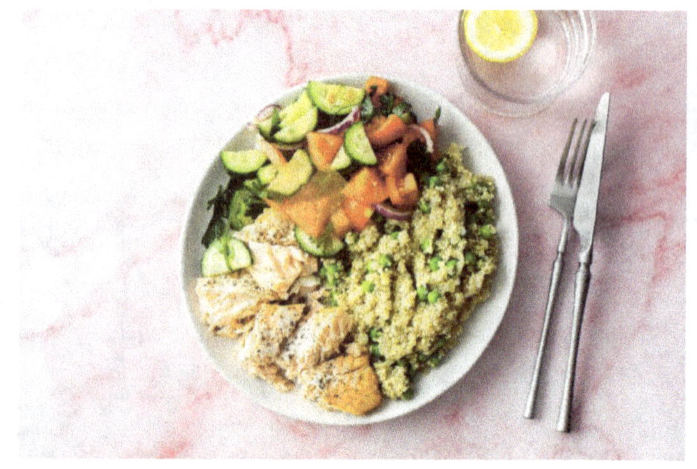

Instructions:

1. Prepare Quinoa:

Rinse the quinoa in cold water through a fine-mesh sieve until it is clear.

In a medium saucepan, heat 2 cups of water to a boil. Combine the rinsed quinoa with a teaspoon of salt. Reduce the heat to low, cover, and let simmer for about 15 minutes, or until the quinoa is cooked and the water has been absorbed. Remove from the heat and allow to settle for 5 minutes, covered. Fluff with a fork.

2. Prepare the steamed vegetables:

Steam the mixed veggies in a steamer basket over a pot of boiling water for 5-7 minutes, or until tender but crisp. Remove from the heat and put aside.

3. Cook the salmon:

Season the salmon fillets with salt, pepper, and any dry herbs you're using.

In a large skillet, warm 1 tablespoon olive oil over medium-high heat. Cook the salmon fillets in the skillet, skin side down if any skin remains, for about 4-5 minutes on each side, or until cooked through and easily flaked with a fork. Remove from the skillet and set aside.

4. Prepare the Lemon Garlic Sauce:

In the same skillet, warm the remaining tablespoon of olive oil over medium heat. Add the minced garlic and simmer for about 1 minute, or until fragrant. Take care not to burn the garlic.

Add the lemon juice to the skillet, scraping off any browned bits from the bottom. Cook for another minute to allow the flavours to come together. Remove from heat.

5. Serve: To serve, divide the cooked quinoa across four plates. Serve each plate with steamed veggies and a cooked salmon fillet. Drizzle the lemon garlic sauce on the salmon and vegetables. Garnish with lemon wedges and more herbs if preferred. Serve immediately and enjoy!

Turkey and Vegetable Stir-Fry

Ingredients:

- 1 lb (450g) turkey breast, thinly sliced
- 2 cups broccoli florets
- 1 red bell pepper, thinly sliced
- 1 yellow bell pepper, thinly sliced
- 1 cup sliced mushrooms
- 1 onion, thinly sliced
- 2 cloves garlic, minced
- 2 tablespoons olive oil
- 2 tablespoons low-sodium soy sauce
- 1 tablespoon rice vinegar
- 1 teaspoon honey or maple syrup (optional)
- 1 teaspoon grated ginger
- Salt and pepper to taste
- Cooked brown rice or quinoa for serving (optional)
- Chopped green onions for garnish (optional)
- Sesame seeds for garnish (optional)

Preparation Time: 25 minutes

Quantity: Serves 4

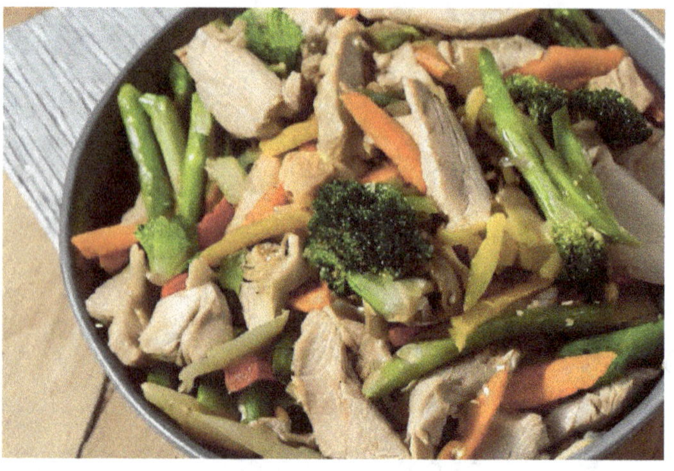

Instructions:

1.   Prepare the ingredients.

Thinly slice the turkey breasts.

Cut the broccoli into florets.

Cut the red and yellow bell peppers, as well as the onion, into thin slices.

Mince the garlic and grate the ginger.

2.   Marinate the turkey.

In a bowl, combine the thinly sliced turkey, soy sauce, rice vinegar, grated ginger, and optional honey or maple syrup. Let it marinade for at least 10 minutes.

3.   Stir-Fry:

Heat the olive oil in a large skillet or wok over medium-high heat.

Add the minced garlic to the skillet and cook for about 30 seconds, until fragrant.

Stir-fry the marinated turkey slices for 3-4 minutes, or until thoroughly done. Remove the turkey from the skillet and set it aside.

4.   Cook the vegetables:

Add extra olive oil to the same skillet if necessary.

Add the broccoli florets, sliced bell peppers, sliced mushrooms, and sliced onion to the skillet.

Stir-fry the vegetables for about 4-5 minutes, or until soft and crisp.

5.   Combine:

Return the cooked turkey to the skillet alongside the veggies.

Stir everything together and cook for a further 1-2 minutes until heated through.

Season with salt and pepper to taste.

6.   Serve:

Serve the turkey and veggie stir fry hot.

Optionally, serve with cooked brown rice or quinoa.

Garnish with chopped green onions and sesame seeds if preferred.

Mediterranean Chickpea Salad

Ingredients:

- 2 cups cooked chickpeas (canned, drained, and rinsed)
- 1 cup cherry tomatoes, halved
- 1 cucumber, diced
- 1 red bell pepper, diced
- 1/4 cup red onion, finely chopped
- 1/4 cup Kalamata olives, pitted and sliced
- 1/4 cup fresh parsley, chopped
- 2 tablespoons extra virgin olive oil
- 2 tablespoons lemon juice
- 1 clove garlic, minced
- Salt and pepper to taste

Prep Time: 15 minutes

Quantity: 4 servings

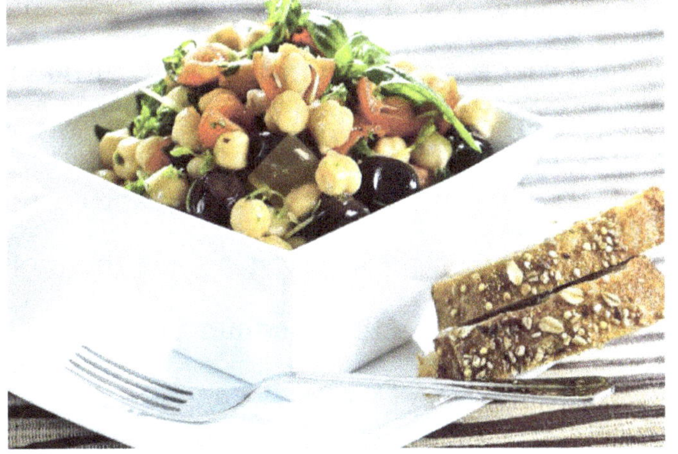

Instructions:

1. In a large mixing bowl, mix together the cooked chickpeas, cherry tomatoes, diced cucumber, diced bell pepper, chopped red onion, sliced Kalamata olives, and chopped parsley.

2. In a small mixing bowl, combine the extra virgin olive oil, lemon juice, minced garlic, salt, and pepper to prepare the dressing.

3. Pour the dressing over the chickpea mixture in a large bowl. Gently toss everything together until well blended and uniformly covered in dressing.

4. Taste and adjust seasoning as needed, adding more salt, pepper, or lemon juice to your taste.

5. After seasoning to your preference, move the Mediterranean Chickpea Salad to a serving dish or individual plates.

6. Serve immediately as a refreshing and nutritious salad, or cover and chill for at

least 30 minutes to allow the flavours to combine before serving.

Grilled Chicken with Roasted Vegetables

Ingredients:

- 4 boneless, skinless chicken breasts
- 2 tablespoons olive oil
- 2 cloves garlic, minced
- 1 teaspoon dried oregano
- 1 teaspoon dried thyme
- Salt and pepper to taste
- 2 zucchinis, sliced
- 1 red bell pepper, sliced
- 1 yellow bell pepper, sliced
- 1 red onion, sliced
- 1 cup cherry tomatoes
- 2 tablespoons balsamic vinegar
- Fresh parsley for garnish

Prep Time: 15 minutes

Cook Time: 25 minutes

Total Time: 40 minutes

Servings: 4

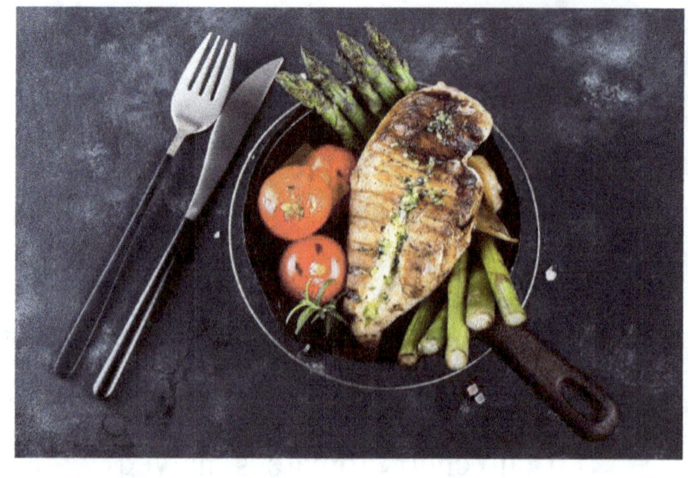

Instructions:

1. Preheat the grill to medium-high heat.

In a small mixing bowl, combine olive oil, minced garlic, dried oregano, dried thyme, salt, and pepper. Mix well.

2. Put the chicken breasts on a shallow dish and coat both sides with the olive oil mixture.

3. Place the chicken breasts on the hot grill and cook for approximately 6-7 minutes per side, or until cooked through and grill marks form. The cooking time may vary based on the thickness of the chicken breasts. Use a meat thermometer to confirm that the interior temperature is 165°F (75°C).

4. While the chicken is cooking, prepare the vegetables. In a large mixing bowl, combine the sliced zucchinis, red bell pepper, yellow bell pepper, red onion, and cherry tomatoes with the remaining olive oil mixture.

5. Place the seasoned vegetables in a single layer on a baking sheet lined with parchment paper.

6. Place the baking sheet under the grill and cook the vegetables for 10-12 minutes, or until soft and slightly browned, stirring halfway through.

7. Remove the chicken from the grill and the veggies from the oven after they have finished cooking.

8. Drizzle balsamic vinegar over the roasted vegetables and mix gently.

9. Serve the grilled chicken beside the roasted veggies, topped with fresh parsley. Enjoy your tasty and nutritious Mind Diet lunch!

Vegetarian Lentil Soup

Ingredients:

- 1 cup dried green or brown lentils, rinsed and drained
- 4 cups vegetable broth
- 1 onion, chopped
- 2 cloves garlic, minced
- 2 carrots, diced
- 2 stalks celery, diced
- 1 can (14.5 oz) diced tomatoes, undrained
- 1 teaspoon ground cumin
- 1 teaspoon smoked paprika
- 1/2 teaspoon dried thyme
- Salt and pepper to taste
- 2 tablespoons olive oil
- 2 cups fresh spinach leaves, chopped
- 1 tablespoon fresh lemon juice
- Fresh parsley, chopped (for garnish)

Prep Time: 15 minutes

Cook Time: 30 minutes

Total Time: 45 minutes

Servings: 4

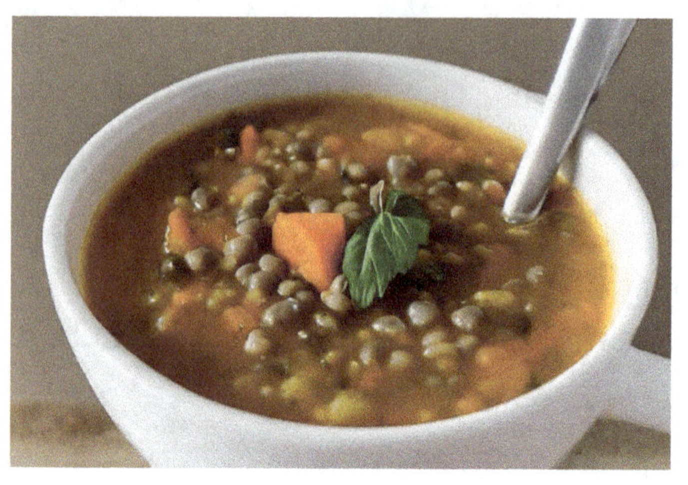

Instructions:

1. In a large pot, heat the olive oil over medium heat. Sauté the chopped onion and garlic until transparent, about 3-4 minutes.

2. Add the diced carrots and celery to the saucepan. Cook for an additional 5 minutes, stirring occasionally.

3. Pour in the vegetable broth, then add the lentils, diced tomatoes (including liquids), ground cumin, smoky paprika, dried thyme, salt, and pepper. Stir thoroughly to mix.

4. Bring the soup to a boil, then reduce the heat to low. Cover and boil for 20-25 minutes, or until the lentils are cooked.

5. Once the lentils are cooked, add the chopped spinach leaves and lemon juice. Cook for an additional 2-3 minutes, until the spinach has wilted.

6. Taste and adjust the seasoning as needed. Add extra salt and pepper to taste.

7. Serve hot and sprinkle with freshly chopped parsley. Enjoy this hearty and healthy vegetarian lentil soup, which is ideal for the Mind Diet and contains plenty of fibre and nutrients.

Baked Cod with Roasted Brussels Sprouts

Ingredients:

- 4 pieces of fresh cod fillets (about 6 ounces each)
- 1 pound Brussels sprouts, trimmed and halved
- 2 tablespoons olive oil
- 2 cloves garlic, minced

- ■ 1 teaspoon lemon zest
- ■ 1 tablespoon lemon juice
- ■ 1 teaspoon dried thyme
- ■ Salt and pepper to taste

Preparation Time: 10 minutes

Cooking Time: 25 minutes

Quantity: Serves 4

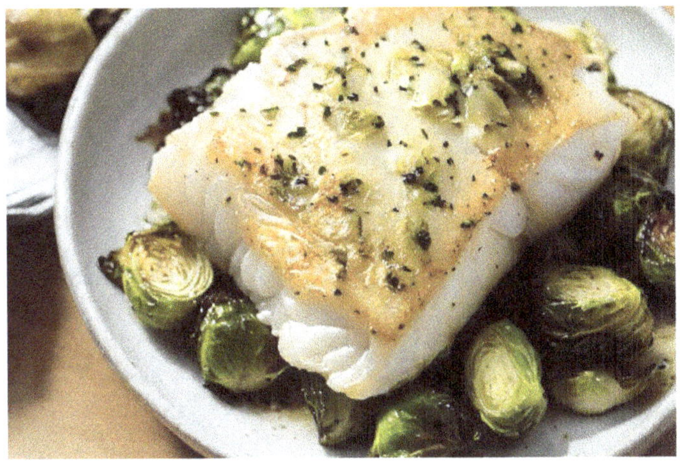

Instructions:

1. Preheat the oven to 400 °F (200 °C). Arrange the halved Brussels sprouts on a baking sheet. Drizzle with 1 tablespoon olive oil, season with salt and pepper, and toss until evenly coated. Spread them out into a single layer.

2. Roast the Brussels sprouts in the preheated oven for 20-25 minutes, or until tender and lightly browned. Stir halfway through.

3. While the Brussels sprouts roast, prepare the cod. Pat the cod fillets dry using paper towels before placing them on another baking sheet coated with parchment paper.

4. In a small bowl, combine the minced garlic, lemon zest, lemon juice, dried thyme, and the remaining tablespoon olive oil. Season the cod fillets with salt and pepper, then brush the garlic and lemon mixture over them.

5. When the Brussels sprouts are almost done, place the baking sheet with the cod in the oven for 12-15 minutes, or until the fish is opaque and readily flaked with a fork.

6. Serve the baked cod with roasted Brussels sprouts.

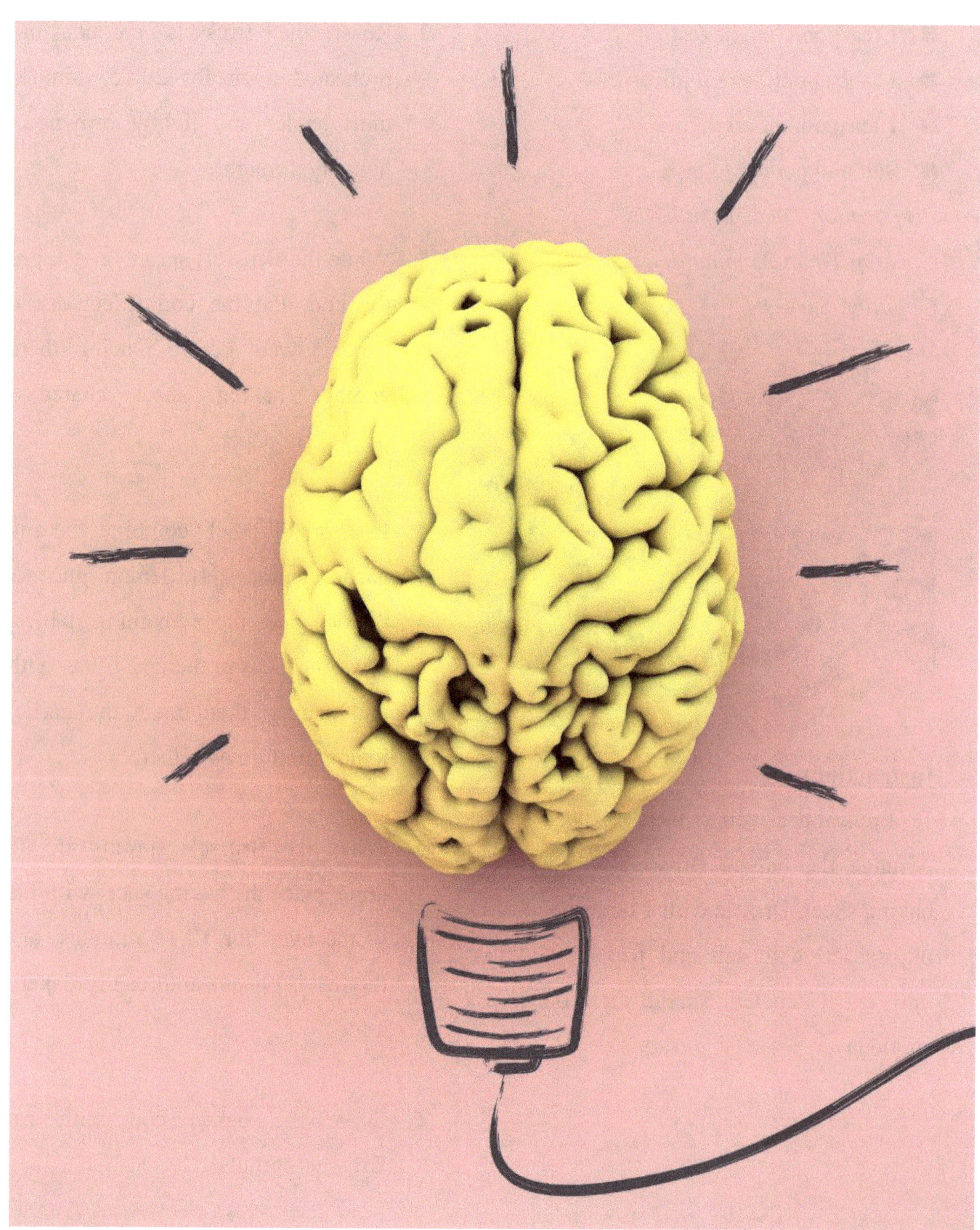

HEALTHY SNACKS FOR MINDFUL MUNCHING

Crunchy Roasted Chickpeas

Ingredients:

- 2 cans (15 ounces each) chickpeas (garbanzo beans), drained and rinsed
- 2 tablespoons olive oil
- 1 teaspoon paprika
- 1 teaspoon garlic powder
- 1/2 teaspoon cumin
- 1/2 teaspoon salt
- 1/4 teaspoon black pepper

Prep Time: 5 minutes
Cook Time: 35 minutes
Total Time: 40 minutes
Quantity: Serves 4

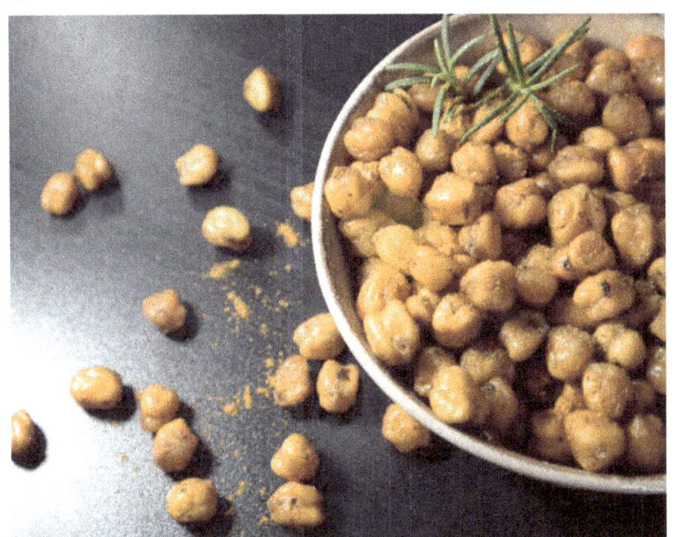

Instructions:

1. Preheat your oven to 400 degrees Fahrenheit (200 degrees Celsius). Line a baking sheet with parchment or aluminium foil.

2. Dry Chickpeas: After draining and rinsing, pat them dry with a clean kitchen towel or paper towels. Keeping them dry will help them crisp up more in the oven.

3. Season chickpeas: In a mixing bowl, combine olive oil, paprika, garlic powder, cumin, salt, and black pepper. Toss until the chickpeas are well covered in the seasonings.

4. Spread the seasoned chickpeas evenly on the prepared baking sheet. Make sure they're equally spaced to ensure even roasting.

5. Roast Chickpeas: Place the baking sheet in the preheated oven and roast for 35

minutes, or until golden brown and crispy. Shake the baking sheet halfway during the cooking time to ensure an even roast.

6. Cool and Serve: After roasting the chickpeas, take them from the oven and let them cool somewhat before serving. They will continue to crisp as they cool. Serve as a crunchy snack or as a garnish on salads or grain bowls.

7. Storage: Keep any leftover crunchy roasted chickpeas in an airtight container at room temperature for up to three days. Enjoy them as a nutritious snack whenever you have a craving!

Blueberry Walnut Yogurt Parfait

Ingredients:

- 1 cup low-fat Greek yogurt
- 1/2 cup fresh blueberries
- 1/4 cup chopped walnuts
- 1 tablespoon honey (optional)
- 1 teaspoon ground flaxseed (optional)

Prep Time: 10 minutes

Quantity: 1 serving

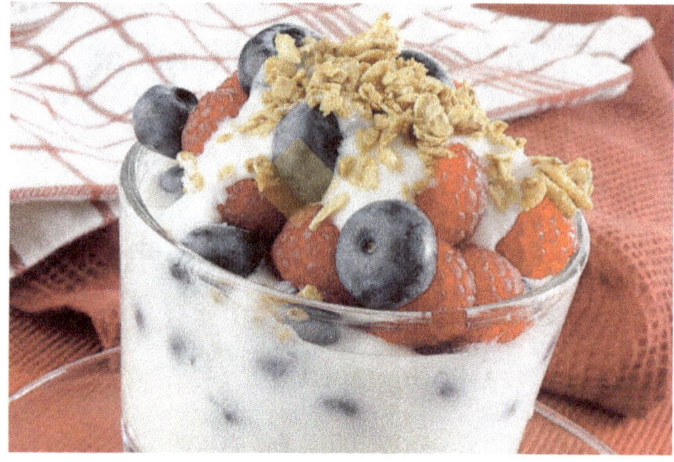

Instructions:

1. Start by gathering all of your ingredients.

2. In a small bowl or glass, place half of the Greek yoghurt.

3. Place half of the fresh blueberries on top of the yoghurt layer.

4. Distribute half of the chopped walnuts evenly over the blueberries.

5. Repeat layering with the remaining yoghurt, blueberries, and walnuts.

6. For more sweetness, drizzle honey over the top.

7. Sprinkle ground flaxseed over the final layer for added nutritional value.

8. Serve immediately, or chill until ready to eat.

9. Enjoy this tasty and nutritious Blueberry Walnut Yoghurt Parfait

Avocado Toast with Tomato

Ingredients:

- 2 ripe avocados
- 4 slices of whole grain bread
- 2 medium-sized tomatoes, thinly sliced
- 1 lemon
- Salt and pepper to taste
- Red pepper flakes (optional)
- Fresh parsley or cilantro for garnish (optional)

Preparation Time: 10 minutes

Quantity: Makes 2 servings

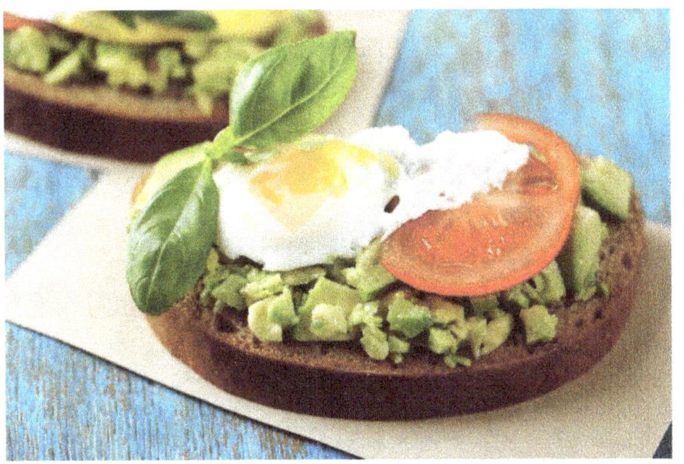

Instructions:

1. Prepare the Avocados: Cut them in half and remove the pits. Scoop the avocado flesh into a bowl.

2. Mash the Avocado: With a fork, mash the avocado till the desired consistency is achieved. Mash lightly to achieve a thick texture. Mash thoroughly to achieve a smoother spread.

3. Season the Avocado: Squeeze half a lemon's juice over the mashed avocado. Add salt and pepper to taste. Mix thoroughly to mix. Adjust the seasoning as needed.

4. Toast the whole grain bread till golden brown and crispy.

5. Assemble the Toast: Spread the mashed avocado evenly on each slice of toasted bread.

6. Add Tomato Slices: Top the avocado spread with thinly sliced tomatoes.

7. Season again (optional): Add red pepper flakes to the tomatoes for flavour and a bit of heat.

8. Garnish (optional): Add fresh parsley or cilantro leaves for a burst of colour and freshness.

9. Serve the avocado toast immediately, while the bread is still warm. Enjoy as a healthy and tasty snack or light supper.

Trail Mix with Dark Chocolate

Ingredients:

- 1 cup almonds, unsalted
- 1 cup walnuts, unsalted
- 1 cup dried blueberries
- 1 cup dried cranberries
- 1 cup dark chocolate chips (at least 70% cocoa)

Preparation Time: 10 minutes

Quantity: Approximately 5 cups of trail mix

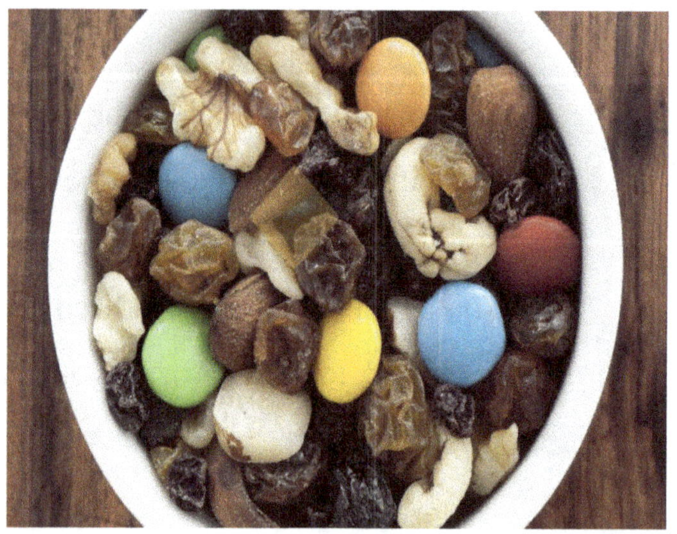

Instructions:

1. Prepare the Ingredients: Gather all of the ingredients in the proper quantities. Make sure the nuts are unsalted and the chocolate chips are dark chocolate with at least 70% cacao.

2. Chop Nuts (Optional): If wanted, chop the almonds and walnuts into smaller pieces with a knife or food processor. This stage is optional and based on personal preference.

3. Ingredients: In a large mixing bowl, add almonds, walnuts, dried blueberries, dried cranberries, and dark chocolate chips. Mix thoroughly so that the ingredients are uniformly distributed.

4. To store the trail mix, transfer it to an airtight container or resealable bags. Make sure to keep it in a cool, dry place away from sunshine.

5. Enjoy Mindfully: For a quick and healthy snack, take a handful of this trail mix.

Spinach and Feta Stuffed Mushrooms

Ingredients:

- 12 large mushrooms, cleaned and stems removed
- 2 cups fresh spinach, chopped
- 1/2 cup crumbled feta cheese
- 1/4 cup diced onion
- 2 cloves garlic, minced
- 1 tablespoon olive oil
- Salt and pepper to taste
- Cooking spray or additional olive oil for greasing

Prep Time: 15 minutes

Quantity: Makes 12 stuffed mushrooms

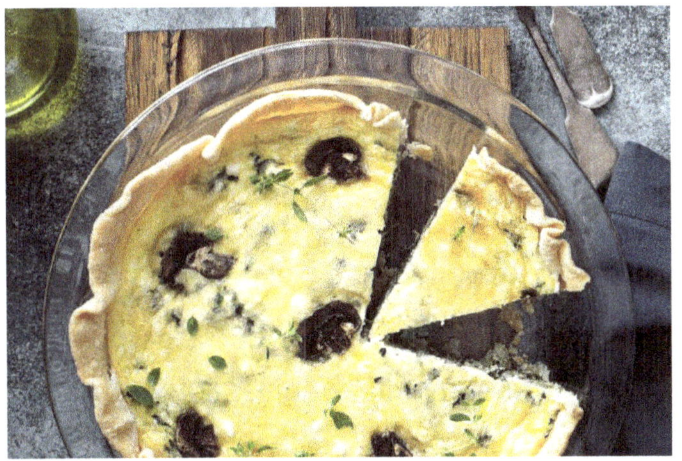

Instructions:

1. Preheat the oven to 375°F (190° C).

2. In a skillet, heat the olive oil over medium heat. Combine the diced onion and minced garlic. Sauté until the onions are transparent and fragrant, which should take around 2-3 minutes.

3. Add the chopped spinach to the skillet. Cook for an additional 2-3 minutes, or until the spinach has wilted. Remove from heat and allow it cool slightly.

4. In a mixing bowl, combine the cooked spinach and crumbled feta cheese. Season with salt and pepper to taste. Mix well.

5. Remove the mushrooms' stems and clean them thoroughly. Coat a baking dish with cooking spray or olive oil.

6. Stuff each mushroom cap with a spoonful of the spinach and feta mixture, gently pressing it in.

7. Place the stuffed mushrooms in the prepared baking dish. If there is any remaining filling, sprinkle it over the mushrooms.

8. Bake in the preheated oven for 15-20 inutes, or until the mushrooms are soft and the filling is thoroughly heated.

9. Once finished, remove from the oven and allow to cool slightly before serving.

Quinoa Salad with Vegetables

- **Ingredients:**1 cup quinoa, rinsed
- 2 cups water or vegetable broth
- 1 cucumber, diced
- 1 bell pepper (any color), diced
- 1 cup cherry tomatoes, halved
- 1/4 cup red onion, finely chopped
- 1/4 cup fresh parsley, chopped
- 1/4 cup fresh mint leaves, chopped
- 1/4 cup black olives, sliced (optional)
- 1/4 cup feta cheese, crumbled (optional)
- Salt and pepper to taste

Dressing:

- 1/4 cup extra virgin olive oil
- 2 tablespoons lemon juice
- 1 clove garlic, minced
- 1 teaspoon Dijon mustard
- 1/2 teaspoon honey or maple syrup
- Salt and pepper to taste

Prep Time: 15 minutes

Quantity: Serves 4

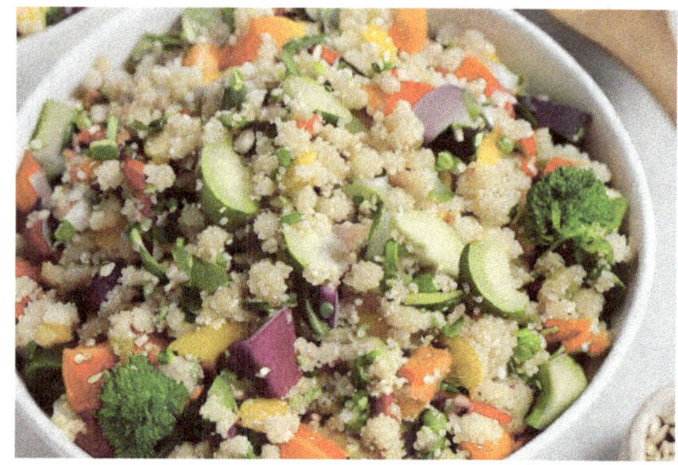

Instructions:

1. To prepare the quinoa, blend it with water or vegetable broth in a medium pot. Bring to a boil, then reduce to a low heat, cover, and cook for 15 minutes, or until the quinoa is soft and the liquid is absorbed. Remove from heat and cover for 5 minutes. Fluff with a fork and allow to cool to room temperature.

2. In a small mixing bowl, combine the dressing ingredients: olive oil, lemon juice, chopped garlic, Dijon mustard, honey or maple syrup, salt, and pepper. Set aside.

3. In a large mixing bowl, mix together the cooked quinoa, diced cucumber, diced bell pepper, cherry tomatoes, sliced red onion, chopped parsley, chopped mint leaves, black olives (if using), and crumbled feta cheese.

4. Pour the dressing over the quinoa and veggie combination. Gently toss everything to provide a uniform coating.

5. Taste and adjust seasoning with salt and pepper as needed.

6. Serve immediately or chill for at least 30 minutes to let the flavours mingle before serving.

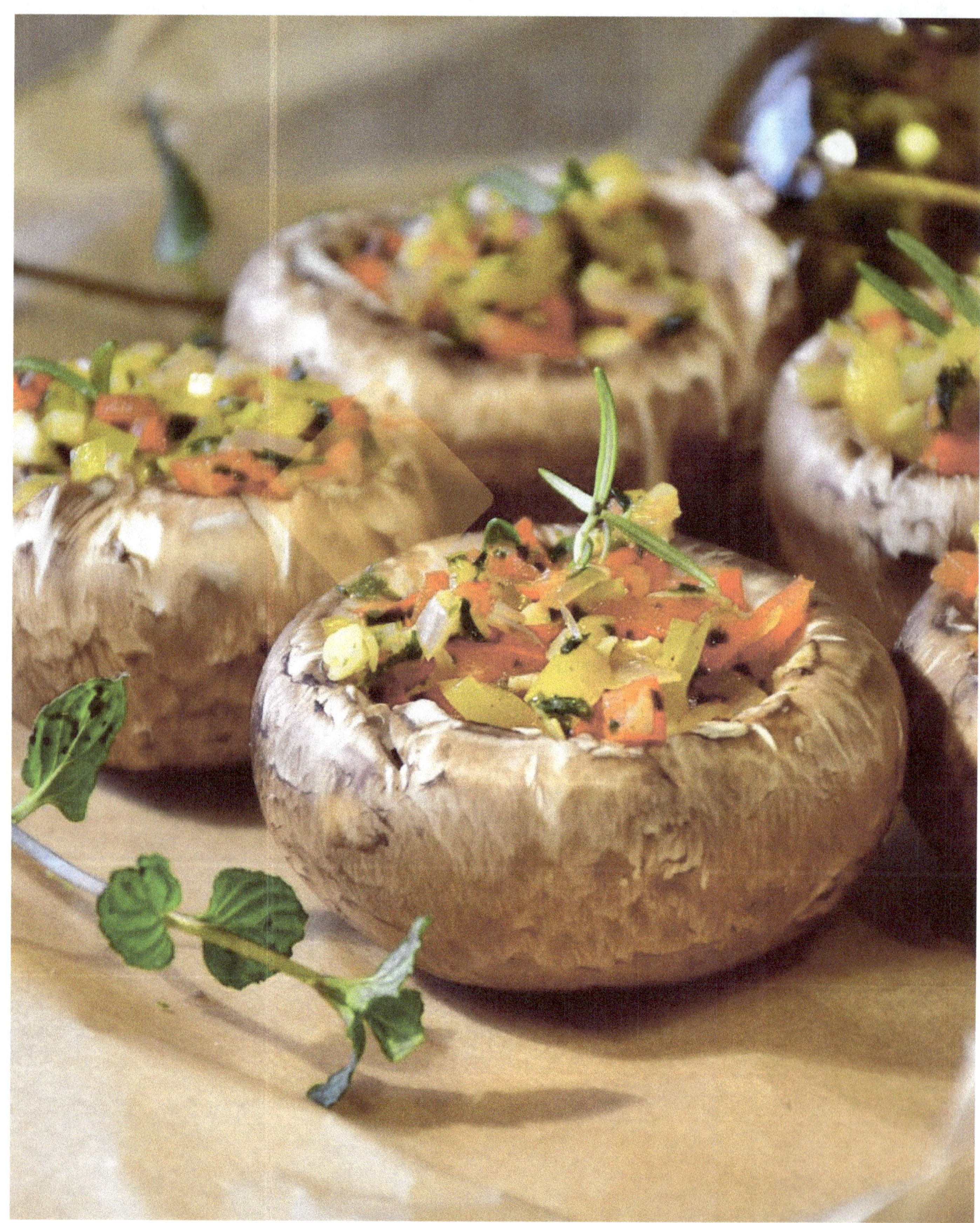

SATISFYING SWEET TREATS

Dark Chocolate Berry Bark

Ingredients:

- 200g dark chocolate (70% cocoa or higher), chopped
- 1 cup mixed berries (such as raspberries, blueberries, and strawberries), washed and dried
- 1/4 cup unsalted almonds, chopped
- 1 tablespoon chia seeds
- 1 tablespoon unsweetened shredded coconut

Prep Time: 15 minutes

Quantity: Makes about 12 servings

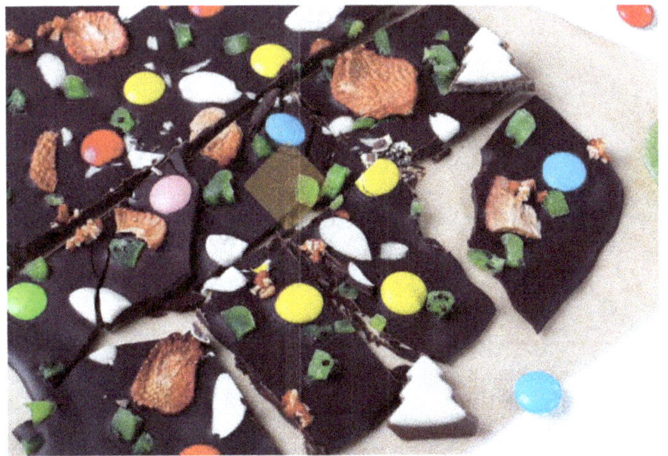

Instructions:

1. Prepare a Baking Sheet: Line a baking sheet with parchment paper and set it aside.

2. Melt the Chocolate: Place the chopped dark chocolate in a microwave-safe bowl. Microwave in 30-second intervals, stirring in between, until the chocolate is completely melted and smooth. Alternatively, you can melt the chocolate using a double boiler on the stovetop.

3. Spread the Chocolate: Pour the melted chocolate onto the prepared baking sheet. Use a spatula to spread it out evenly into a rectangle, about 1/4 inch thick.

4. Add Berries and Nuts: Sprinkle the mixed berries, chopped almonds, chia seeds, and shredded coconut evenly over the melted chocolate.

5. Chill in the Refrigerator: Place the baking sheet in the refrigerator and chill for about 1 hour, or until the chocolate has completely hardened.

6. Break into Pieces: Once the chocolate has hardened, remove the baking sheet from the refrigerator. Use your hands or a knife to break the bark into pieces of your desired size.

7. Serve or Store: Serve the dark chocolate berry bark immediately, or store it in an airtight container in the refrigerator for up to one week. Enjoy as a delicious and satisfying treat!

Coconut Chia Pudding

Ingredients:

- 1 cup coconut milk
- 1/4 cup chia seeds
- 1 tablespoon honey or maple syrup (optional)
- 1/2 teaspoon vanilla extract
- 1/4 cup unsweetened shredded coconut
- Fresh berries for topping (optional)
- Chopped nuts for topping (optional)

Prep Time: 5 minutes
Quantity: Serves 2

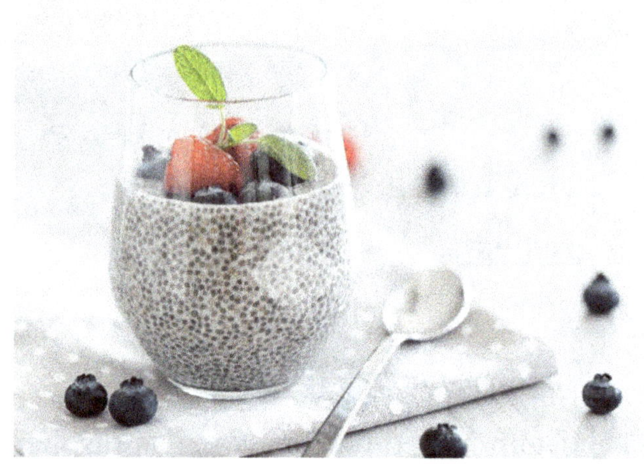

Instructions:

1. In a mixing dish, combine the coconut milk, chia seeds, honey or maple syrup (if using), vanilla essence, and coconut flakes. Stir well to fully blend all of the ingredients.

2. Cover the bowl with plastic wrap or put the mixture in an airtight container.

3. Refrigerate the mixture for at least 2 hours, preferably overnight. This causes the chia seeds to absorb liquid and form a pudding-like consistency.

4. After chilling, mix the pudding to spread the chia seeds evenly.

5. Divide the pudding among serving bowls or glasses.

6. If preferred, top with chopped nuts and fresh berries.

7. Serve chilled and enjoy this delicious and nutritious coconut chia pudding as part of your Mind Diet.

Baked Apples with Cinnamon and Walnuts

Ingredients:

- 4 medium-sized apples (such as Granny Smith or Honeycrisp)
- 1/4 cup chopped walnuts
- 2 tablespoons honey or maple syrup
- 1 teaspoon ground cinnamon
- 1/4 teaspoon ground nutmeg
- 1 tablespoon melted coconut oil or butter (optional)

Prep Time: 10 minutes
Quantity: Serves 4

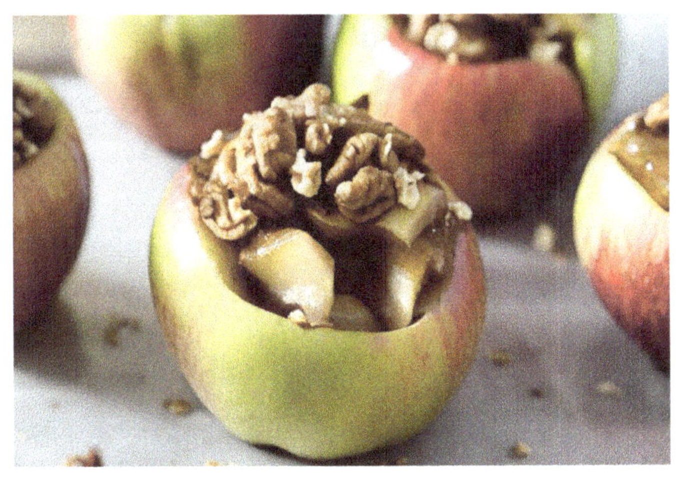

Instructions:

1. Preheat the oven to 375°F (190° C).

2. Wash the apples thoroughly, then pat them dry with a clean dish towel.

3. Core the apples with an apple corer or a sharp knife, removing the seeds and forming a well in the centre.

4. In a small bowl, blend the chopped walnuts, honey or maple syrup, ground cinnamon, and ground nutmeg until thoroughly incorporated.

5. Stuff each cored apple with the walnut mixture, distributing it evenly.

6. Drizzle melted coconut oil or butter over the filled apples.

7. Place the stuffed apples in a baking dish or on a baking sheet covered with parchment paper.

8. Bake in a preheated oven for 25-30 minutes, or until the apples are soft and the filling is bubbling.

9. Once baked, remove the apples from the oven and allow to cool slightly before serving.

10. Optional toppings include a spoonful of Greek yoghurt and a sprinkling of cinnamon.

Frozen Banana Bites

Ingredients:

- 2 ripe bananas
- 1/4 cup natural peanut butter or almond butter (no added sugar)
- 1/4 cup dark chocolate chips (at least 70% cocoa)
- 2 tablespoons unsweetened shredded coconut (optional)
- 2 tablespoons chopped nuts (optional, such as almonds, walnuts, or pecans)

Prep Time: 15 minutes

Quantity: Makes about 12 bites

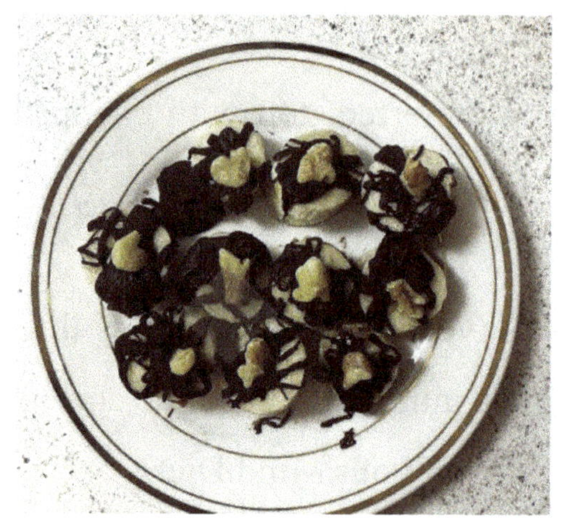

Instructions:

1. Peel the bananas and cut them into thick slices of about 1/2 inch each. Place the banana slices on a parchment-lined baking sheet or platter.

2. In a small microwave-safe bowl, heat the peanut butter for about 20-30 seconds until it softens and becomes easier to deal with.

3. With a knife or spoon, spread a thin coating of melted peanut butter on one side of each banana slice.

4. Place half of the banana slices in pairs, peanut butter side up, on the prepared baking sheet or dish.

5. Place the other half of the banana slices on top of the peanut butter, forming mini banana sandwiches.

6. In another small microwave-safe bowl, microwave the dark chocolate chips for 20-30 seconds, stirring in between, until smooth and melted.

7. Dip each banana sandwich halfway into the melted chocolate, then return to the parchment-lined baking sheet or plate.

8. Optional: Before the melted chocolate solidifies, sprinkle it with shredded coconut or chopped nuts.

9. Once all of the banana sandwiches have been dipped and coated, place the baking sheet or plate in the freezer for at least 2 hours, or until the chocolate has set and the banana bites are solidly frozen.

10. Once frozen, place the banana bites in an airtight container or freezer bag to store.

Blueberry Oatmeal Muffins

Ingredients:

- 1 1/2 cups all-purpose flour
- 1 cup rolled oats
- 1/2 cup granulated sugar
- 2 teaspoons baking powder
- 1/2 teaspoon baking soda
- 1/2 teaspoon salt
- 1 cup plain yogurt
- 1/4 cup milk
- 1/4 cup vegetable oil
- 2 large eggs
- 1 teaspoon vanilla extract
- 1 1/2 cups fresh or frozen blueberries

Preparation Time:15 minutes

Cook: 20 minutes

Total: 35 minutes

Quantity: Makes about 12 muffins

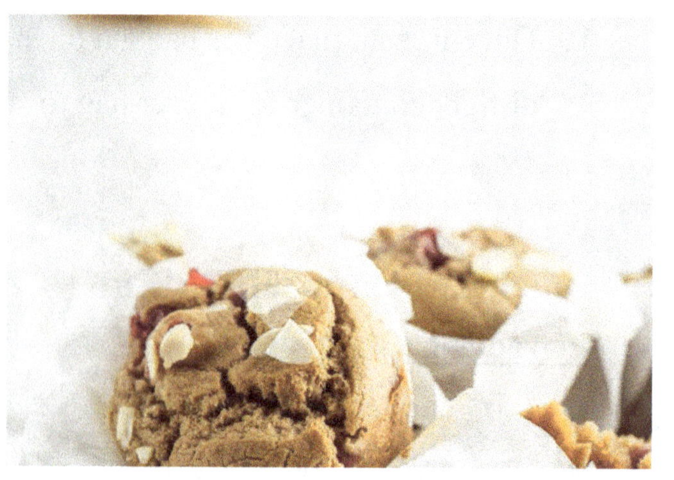

Instructions:

1. Preheat the oven to 375°F (190° C). Grease or line a muffin tray with paper liners.

2. In a large mixing basin, mix together the flour, rolled oats, sugar, baking powder, baking soda, and salt. Stir until thoroughly combined.

3. In a separate bowl, whisk together the yoghurt, milk, vegetable oil, eggs, and vanilla extract until smooth.

4. Pour the wet ingredients into the dry mixture. Stir just until mixed. Don't overmix the batter; it should be somewhat lumpy.

5. Gently fold in the blueberries, taking care not to bruise them.

6. Spoon the batter into the muffin cups, filling them about 3/4 full.

7. Bake the muffins for 18-20 minutes, or until golden brown and a toothpick inserted in the centre comes out clean.

8. Remove the muffins from the oven and cool in the tray for 5 minutes before transferring to a wire rack to finish cooling.

Dark Chocolate Avocado Brownies
Ingredients:

- 2 ripe avocados
- 1/2 cup dark chocolate chips
- 1/2 cup cocoa powder
- 1/2 cup honey or maple syrup
- 2 eggs
- 1 teaspoon vanilla extract
- 1/2 teaspoon baking powder
- Pinch of salt

Prep Time: 15 minutes

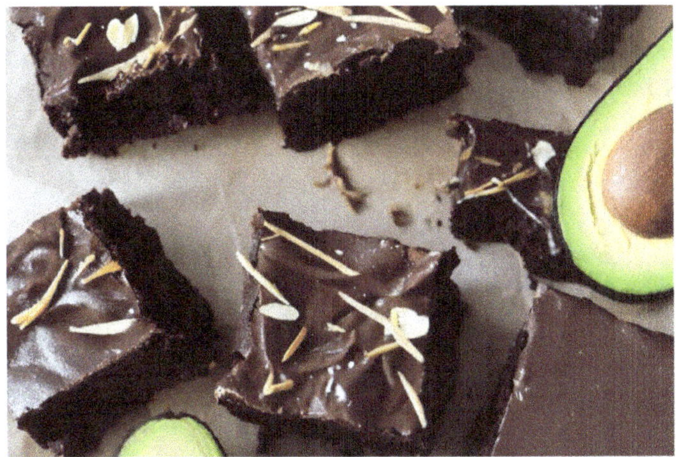

Quantity: Makes about 12 brownies

Instructions:

1. Preheat the oven to 350°F (175° C). Grease a baking pan and leave aside.

2. In a microwave-safe bowl, melt the dark chocolate chips until smooth, stirring every 30 seconds.

3. In a food processor or blender, add ripe avocados, melted chocolate, cocoa powder, honey (or maple syrup), eggs, vanilla extract, baking powder, and salt. Blend until smooth.

4. Pour the mixture onto the prepared baking pan and distribute evenly.

5. Bake in a preheated oven for 25-30 minutes, or until a toothpick inserted in the centre comes out clean.

6. Let the brownies cool before slicing and serving. Enjoy these tasty and nutritious Dark Chocolate Avocado Brownies!

Coconut Almond Energy Balls

Ingredients:

- 1 cup almonds
- 1 cup shredded coconut
- 1/2 cup dates, pitted
- 2 tablespoons almond butter
- 1 tablespoon honey

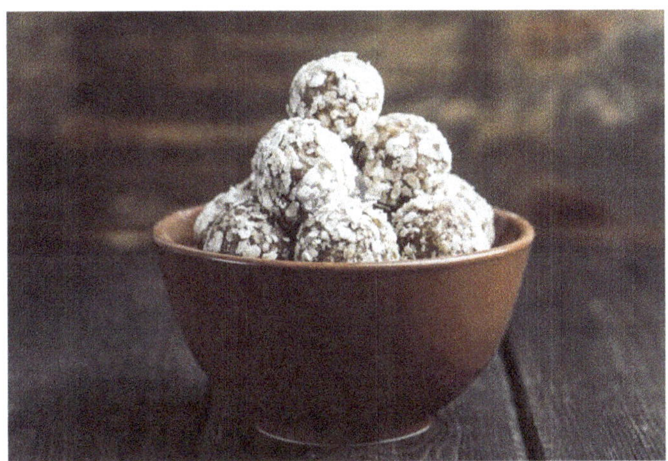

- 1/2 teaspoon vanilla extract
- Pinch of salt

Prep Time: 15 minutes

Quantity: Makes about 12 energy balls

Instructions:

1. Put almonds in a food processor and pulse until finely chopped.

2. Add the shredded coconut, dates, almond butter, honey, vanilla essence, and salt to the food processor.

3. Mix the ingredients until they form a sticky dough.

4. Scoop out about a tablespoon of the mixture and roll it into balls with your palms.

5. Repeat with the remaining mixture.

6. Keep the energy balls in an airtight jar in the refrigerator for up to a week.

7. Enjoy this quick and healthy snack!

Berry Yogurt Parfait

Ingredients:

- 1 cup Greek yogurt
- 1 cup mixed berries (such as strawberries, blueberries, raspberries)
- 1/2 cup granola
- Honey or maple syrup (optional)
- Fresh mint leaves for garnish (optional)

Prep Time: 5 minutes

Quantity: 2 servings

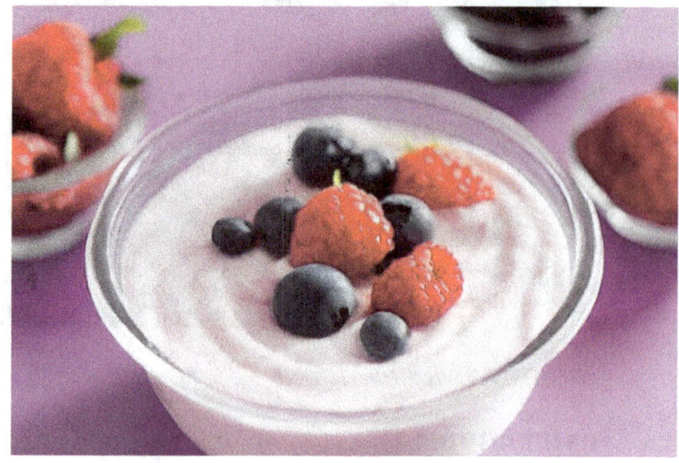

Instruction:

1. In two serving glasses or bowls, put a layer of Greek yoghurt on the bottom.

2. Place a layer of mixed berries on top of the yoghurt.

3. Sprinkle granola over the fruit.

4. Repeat until the glasses are full, finishing with a layer of granola on top.

5. If desired, drizzle the top with honey or maple syrup.

6. Garnish with fresh mint leaves.

7. Serve immediately and enjoy!

BEVERAGES FOR BRAIN HEALTH

Green Tea and Lemon Infusion

Ingredients:

- 2 green tea bags
- 1 lemon
- 4 cups of water
- Honey (optional, for sweetness)

Prep Time: 5 minutes

Quantity: 2 servings

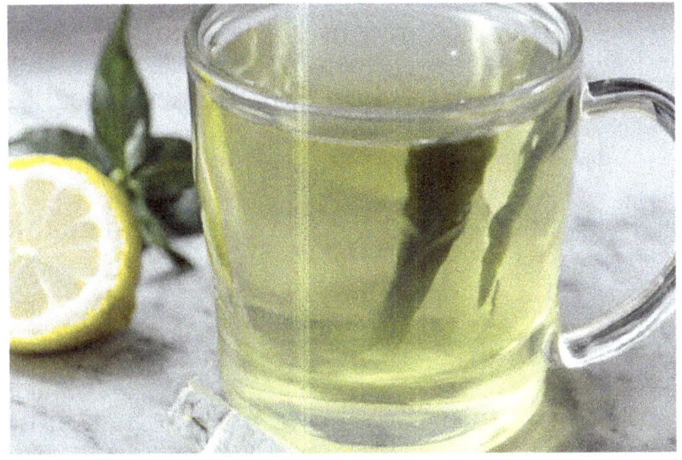

Instructions:

1. Bring 4 cups of water to a boil in a kettle.
2. Cut the lemon into thin pieces.
3. Add the lemon slices to the boiling water.
4. Turn off the heat and steep two green tea bags in the water for three to four minutes.
5. Remove the teabags and lemon slices.
6. Optionally, add honey to taste.
7. Pour the infusion into cups and serve hot, or chill in the refrigerator for a cool beverage. Enjoy!

Berry Blast Smoothie

Ingredients:

- 1 cup mixed berries (strawberries, blueberries, raspberries)
- 1 banana, peeled and sliced
- 1/2 cup Greek yogurt
- 1/2 cup almond milk (or any milk of your choice)
- 1 tablespoon honey (optional)
- Ice cubes (optional)

Prep Time: 5 minutes

Quantity: Makes 2 servings

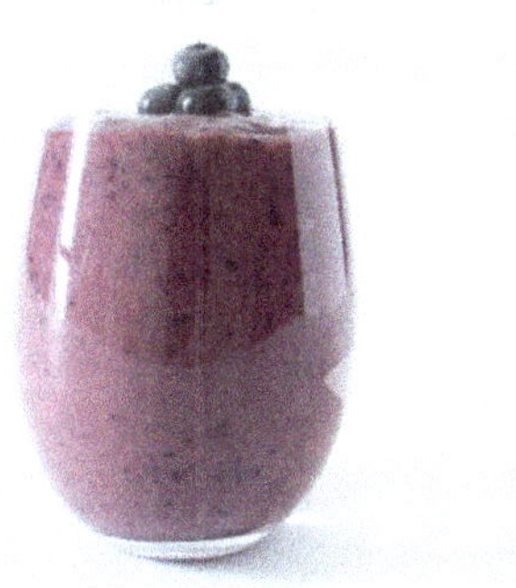

Instructions:

1. Mix the berries, sliced banana, Greek yoghurt, almond milk, and honey (if used) in a blender.

2. Blend until smooth and creamy.

3. If needed, add ice cubes to create a cooler texture and blend again.

4. Pour into glasses and serve immediately. Enjoy your cool Berry Blast Smoothie!

Golden Milk Latte

Ingredients:

- 2 cups of milk (dairy or plant-based)
- 1 teaspoon ground turmeric
- 1/2 teaspoon ground cinnamon
- 1/4 teaspoon ground ginger
- 1 tablespoon honey or maple syrup (adjust to taste)
- 1/2 teaspoon vanilla extract
- A pinch of ground black pepper (optional)

Prep Time: 5 minutes

Quantity: 2 servings

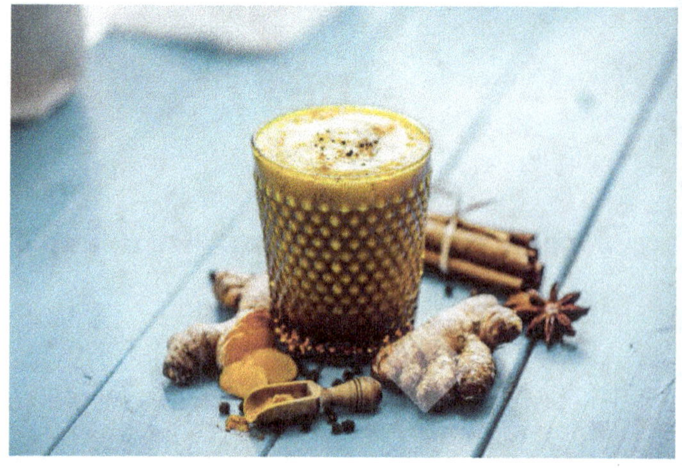

Instructions:

1. In a small saucepan, whisk together milk, turmeric, cinnamon, ginger, honey (or maple syrup), and vanilla extract.

2. Heat the mixture over medium heat until it begins to boil, stirring periodically.

3. Once simmering, drop the heat to low and let it sit for 2-3 minutes to enable the flavours to merge.

4. Remove from the heat and strain the mixture through a fine mesh strainer to remove any remaining spices.

5. Pour the golden milk latte into glasses and serve warm.

6. Sprinkle a teaspoon of black pepper on top before serving for extra flavour. Enjoy your calming and tasty golden milk latte.

Fresh Fruit and Herb Infused Water

Ingredients:

- Assorted fresh fruits (such as berries, citrus fruits, melons, or pineapple)
- Fresh herbs (such as mint, basil, or rosemary)
- Filtered water
- Ice cubes (optional)

Prep Time: 10 minutes

Quantity: 1 pitcher (about 8 cups)

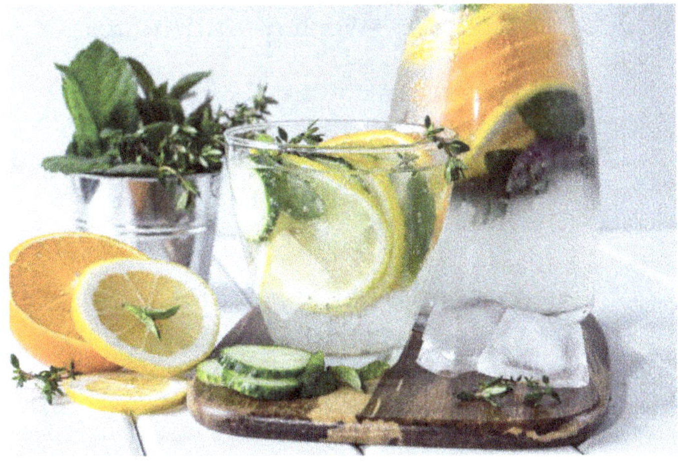

Instructions:

1. Wash fruits and herbs thoroughly with cold water.
2. Slice the fruit into thin rounds or wedges.
3. Tear or lightly bruise the herbs to extract their flavours.
4. Put the cut fruits and torn herbs in a pitcher.
5. Fill the pitcher with purified water.
6. If you want it extra cold, add ice cubes.
7. Stir gently to blend the ingredients.
8. Refrigerate the infused water for at least an hour before serving to allow the flavours to combine.
9. Serve the cool flavoured water over ice.
10. Enjoy the refreshing flavour and hydration!

Blueberry Brain Blast Smoothie:

Ingredients:

- 1 cup blueberries (fresh or frozen)
- 1 ripe banana
- 1/2 cup Greek yogurt
- 1/2 cup almond milk (or any milk of your choice)
- 1 tablespoon honey (optional)
- 1 tablespoon chia seeds (optional)
- Ice cubes (optional)

Prep Time: 5 minutes

Quantity: Makes 2 servings

Instructions:

1. Combine blueberries, banana, Greek yoghurt, almond milk, honey, and chia seeds in a blender.

2. If desired, add a handful of ice cubes to achieve a cooler texture.

3. Blend until smooth and creamy.

4. Pour into glasses and serve immediately.

5. Enjoy your delightful Blueberry Brain Blast Smoothie.

Green Tea Matcha Latte:

Ingredients:

- 1 teaspoon green tea matcha powder
- 1 cup milk (any type, such as cow's milk, almond milk, oat milk, etc.)
- 1 teaspoon honey or sweetener of choice (optional)
- Hot water (for mixing)

Prep Time: 5 minutes

Quantity: 1 serving

Instructions:

1. Heat the milk in a saucepan or microwave until it's hot but not boiling.

2. In a cup, combine the green tea and matcha powder.

3. Pour a little amount of boiling water into the cup containing matcha powder and rapidly whisk until smooth.

4. Pour the heated milk into the matcha mixture and whisk thoroughly.

5. If desired, sweeten with honey or other favourite sweetener.

6. Enjoy your soothing and tasty Green Tea Matcha Latte!

Berry Beet Brain Booster Juice:

Ingredients:

- 1 cup mixed berries (such as strawberries, blueberries, raspberries)
- 1 small beet, peeled and chopped
- 1 medium orange, peeled and segmented
- 1 tablespoon chia seeds
- 1 cup coconut water
- 1 teaspoon honey (optional)

Prep Time: 10 minutes

Quantity: 2 servings

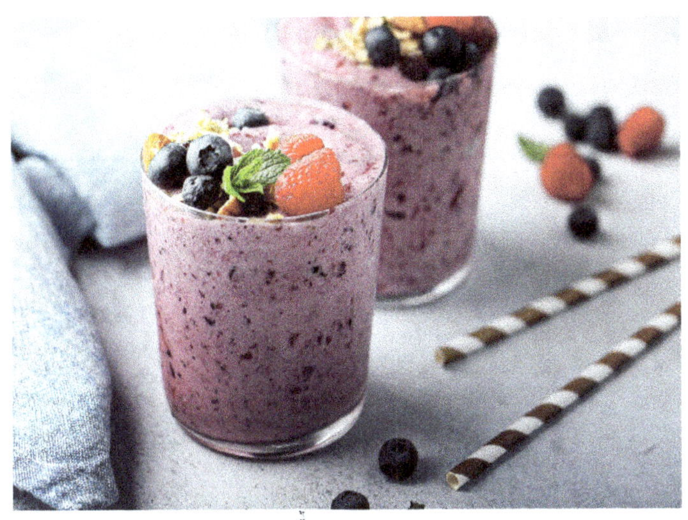

Instructions:

1. Wash all berries well.
2. Peel and cut the beets.
3. Peel and segment an orange.
4. In a blender, combine the mixed berries, sliced beetroot, orange segments, chia seeds, coconut water and honey (if desired).
5. Blend until smooth and thoroughly incorporated.
6. Pour juice into cups and serve immediately.
7. Enjoy your Berry Beet Brain Booster Juice!

Turmeric Golden Milk:

Ingredients:

- 2 cups milk (dairy or plant-based)
- 1 teaspoon ground turmeric
- 1/2 teaspoon ground cinnamon
- 1/4 teaspoon ground ginger
- Pinch of black pepper
- 1-2 teaspoons honey or maple syrup (optional)

Prep Time: 5 minutes

Quantity: Makes 2 servings

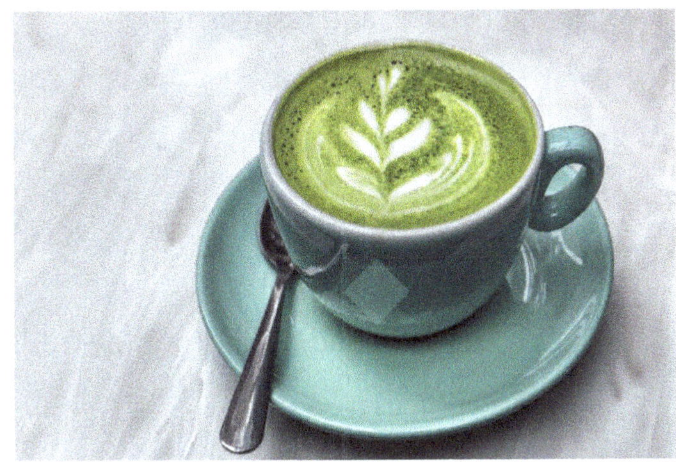

Instructions:

- In a small saucepan, heat the milk over medium heat until it is warm but not boiling.
- Combine the ground turmeric, cinnamon, ginger, and black pepper.

- Whisk the ingredients until thoroughly blended and heated, which should take around 2-3 minutes.
- Remove from the heat and, if preferred, add honey or maple syrup.
- Pour into mugs and serve warm. Enjoy your relaxing turmeric golden milk!

Omega-3 Berry Blast Smoothie:

Ingredients:

- 1 cup mixed berries (such as strawberries, blueberries, and raspberries)
- 1 ripe banana
- 1 tablespoon ground flaxseeds
- 1 tablespoon chia seeds
- 1/2 cup Greek yogurt
- 1/2 cup almond milk (or any milk of your choice)
- 1 tablespoon honey or maple syrup (optional)
- Ice cubes (optional)

Prep Time: 5 minutes

Quantity: Makes 2 servings

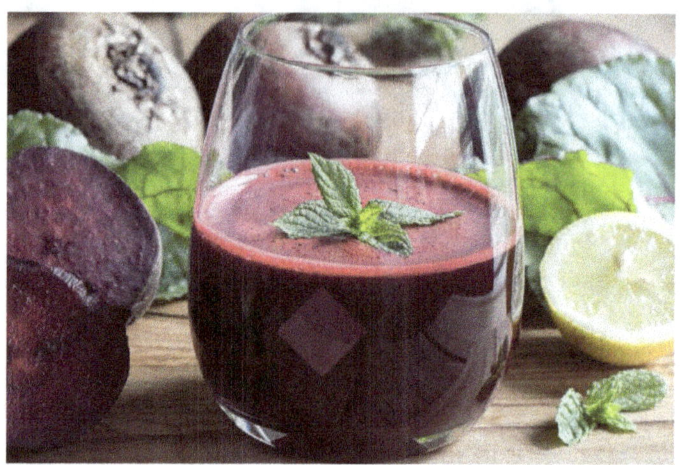

Instructions:

1. Combine all of the ingredients in a blender.
2. Blend until smooth and creamy.
3. If needed, add ice cubes and blend again until the desired consistency is achieved.
4. Pour into cups and drink immediately.

DRESSINGS AND SAUCES

Walnut Pesto:

Ingredients:

- 2 cups fresh basil leaves
- 1/2 cup walnuts, toasted
- 2 cloves garlic
- 1/2 cup grated Parmesan cheese
- 1/2 cup extra virgin olive oil
- Salt and pepper to taste

Prep Time: 10 minutes

Quantity: Makes about 1 cup of walnut pesto

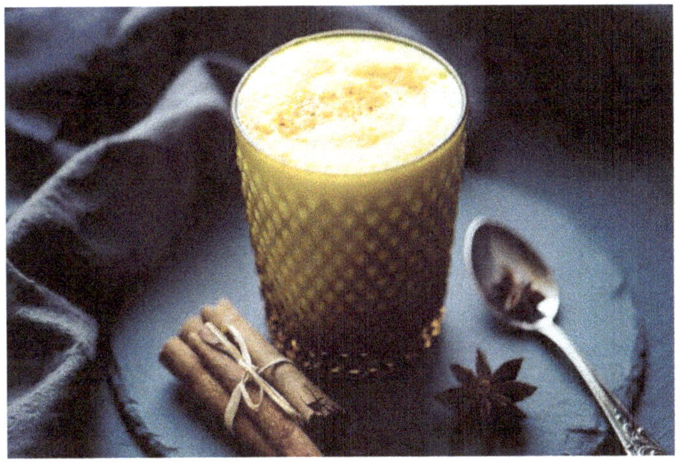

Instructions:

1. In a food processor, combine the basil leaves, roasted walnuts, garlic cloves, and grated Parmesan cheese.

2. Pulse the ingredients until they are finely minced.

3. While the food processor is running, carefully pour in the olive oil until the mixture reaches a smooth consistency.

4. Season with salt and pepper to taste, then pulse a couple more times to blend.

5. Transfer the walnut pesto to a jar or airtight container and refrigerate until ready to use. Enjoy!

Avocado Yogurt Dressing:

Ingredients:

- 1 ripe avocado
- 1/2 cup plain yogurt
- 2 tablespoons lime juice
- 1 clove garlic, minced
- Salt and pepper to taste

Prep Time: 5 minutes

Quantity: Makes about 1 cup of dressing

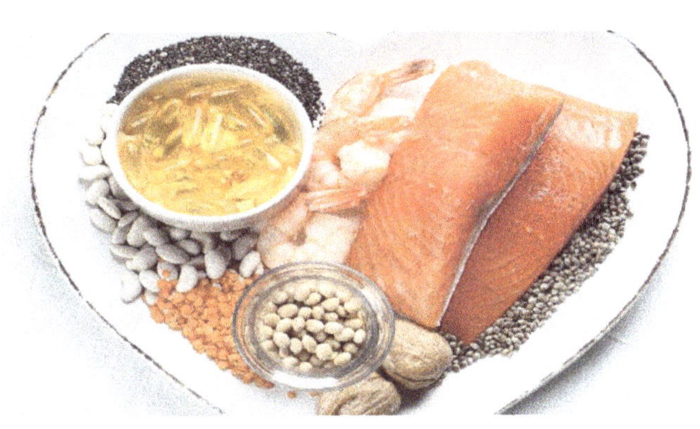

<u>**Instructions:**</u>

1. Cut the avocado in halves, remove the pit, and transfer the flesh to a blender or food processor.
2. Add the yoghurt, lime juice, minced garlic, salt, and pepper to a blender.
3. Blend until smooth and creamy, scraping down the sides as necessary.
4. Taste and adjust seasoning as needed.
5. Transfer the dressing to a jar or airtight container and chill until ready to use.
6. Serve over salads, dips, or as a topping for a variety of foods. Enjoy!

Turmeric Tahini Sauce:

<u>**Ingredients:**</u>

- 1/2 cup tahini
- 1/4 cup water
- 2 tablespoons lemon juice
- 1 clove garlic, minced
- 1 teaspoon ground turmeric
- Salt to taste

Prep Time: 5 minutes

Quantity: Approximately 3/4 cup

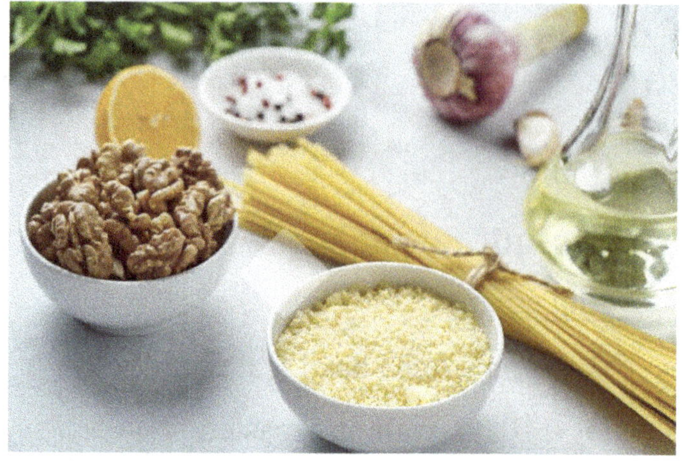

<u>**Instructions:**</u>

1. In a small mixing bowl, combine tahini, water, and lemon juice. Whisk until smooth.
2. Stir in the minced garlic, ground turmeric, and salt.
3. Season to taste.
4. Serve immediately or refrigerate in an airtight container for up to one week.
5. Enjoy as a dip, dressing, or sauce with your favourite foods!

Blueberry Balsamic Vinaigrette:

Ingredients:

- 1 cup fresh blueberries
- 1/4 cup balsamic vinegar
- 2 tablespoons honey
- 1/3 cup olive oil
- Salt and pepper to taste

Prep Time: 5 minutes

Quantity: Makes about 1 cup

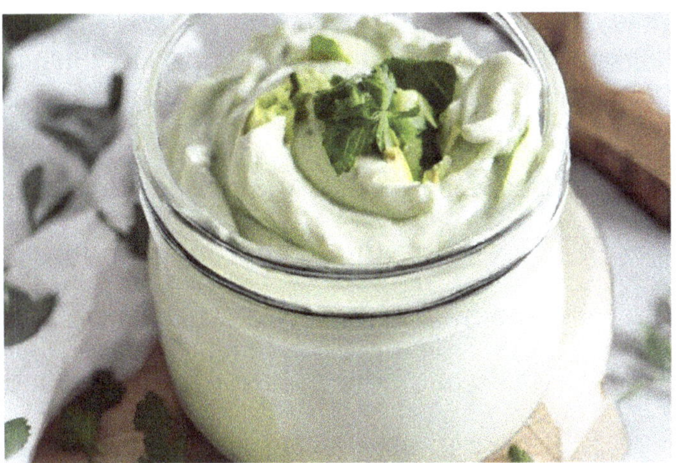

Instructions:

1. In a blender or food processor, combine the blueberries, balsamic vinegar, and honey.
2. Blend until smooth.
3. While combining, carefully sprinkle in the olive oil until it forms an emulsion.
4. Season with salt and pepper to taste.
5. Place the vinaigrette in a jar or container with a lid.
6. Refrigerate for up to one week.
7. Shake thoroughly before serving. Enjoy with salads or as a marinade!

Sesame Ginger Dressing:

Ingredients:

- 1/4 cup soy sauce
- 2 tablespoons sesame oil
- 2 tablespoons rice vinegar
- 1 tablespoon honey
- 1 teaspoon grated ginger
- 1 clove garlic, minced
- 1 tablespoon sesame seeds
- 1/4 cup olive oil

Prep Time: 5 minutes

Quantity: Makes about 3/4 cup of dressing

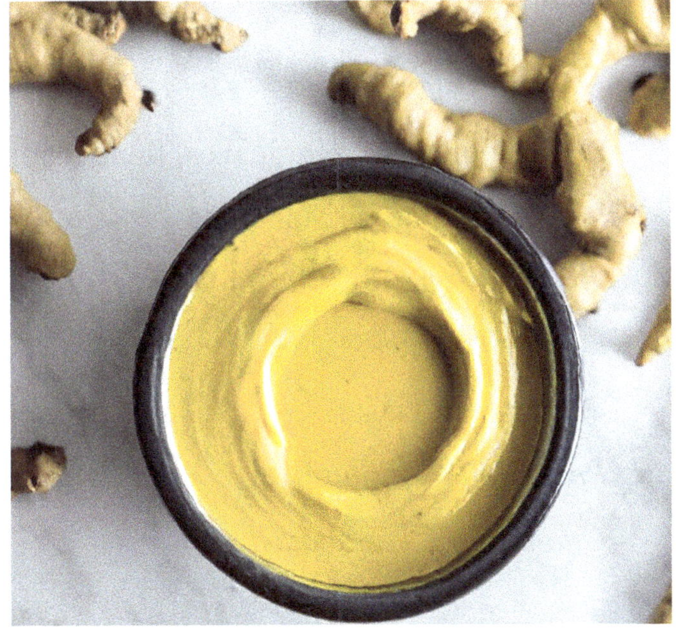

Instructions:

1. In a small mixing bowl, blend soy sauce, sesame oil, rice vinegar, honey, grated ginger, chopped garlic, and sesame seeds until well incorporated.
2. Slowly sprinkle in the olive oil while whisking constantly until the dressing is emulsified.
3. Taste and adjust the seasoning as needed.
4. Refrigerate in an airtight container for up to a week.
5. Shake well before use. Enjoy with salads, grilled veggies, or as a marinade for chicken or tofu.

Minty Yogurt Sauce:

Ingredients:

- 1 cup plain yogurt
- 1/4 cup fresh mint leaves, finely chopped
- 1 tablespoon lemon juice
- 1 clove garlic, minced
- Salt to taste
- Pepper to taste

Prep Time: 5 minutes

Quantity: Makes about 1 cup

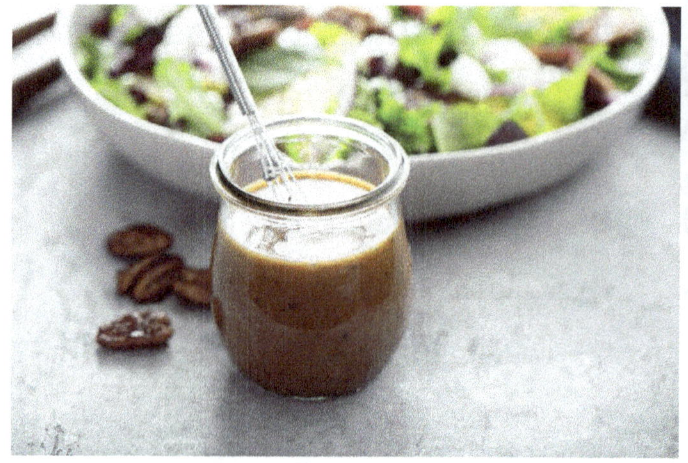

Instructions:

1. In a mixing bowl, add plain yoghurt, finely chopped mint, minced garlic, and lemon juice.
2. Season with salt and pepper to taste.
3. Mix everything thoroughly until it is smooth and evenly distributed.
4. Taste and adjust seasoning as needed.
5. Serve immediately, or chill until ready to use.
6. Enjoy your delicious Minty Yoghurt Sauce as a dip or topping on a variety of foods!

Beet Hummus:

Ingredients:

- 2 medium beets, cooked and peeled
- 1 can (15 oz) chickpeas, drained and rinsed
- 2 cloves garlic, minced
- 3 tablespoons tahini
- 3 tablespoons lemon juice
- 2 tablespoons olive oil
- 1 teaspoon ground cumin
- Salt and pepper to taste
- Water (as needed for consistency)
- Optional garnish: chopped fresh parsley, drizzle of olive oil

Prep Time: 15 minutes
Quantity: Makes about 2 cups of hummus

Instructions:

1. In a food processor, combine the cooked beets, chickpeas, garlic, tahini, lemon juice, olive oil, ground cumin, salt, and pepper.
2. Blend until smooth, scraping the sides of the processor as necessary.
3. If the hummus is too thick, add 1 tablespoon water at a time until the appropriate consistency is achieved.
4. Taste and adjust seasoning as needed.
5. Move the beetroot hummus to a serving bowl.
6. If desired, garnish with chopped fresh parsley and drizzle with olive oil.
7. Serve alongside pita bread, crackers, or veggie sticks.
8. Enjoy this vivid and healthful beetroot hummus!

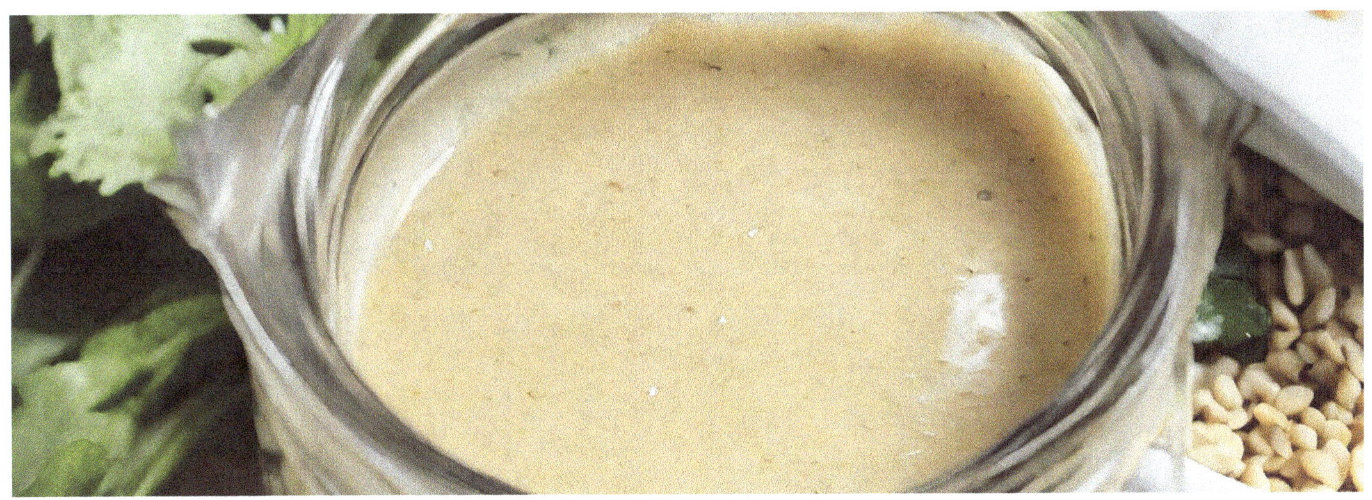

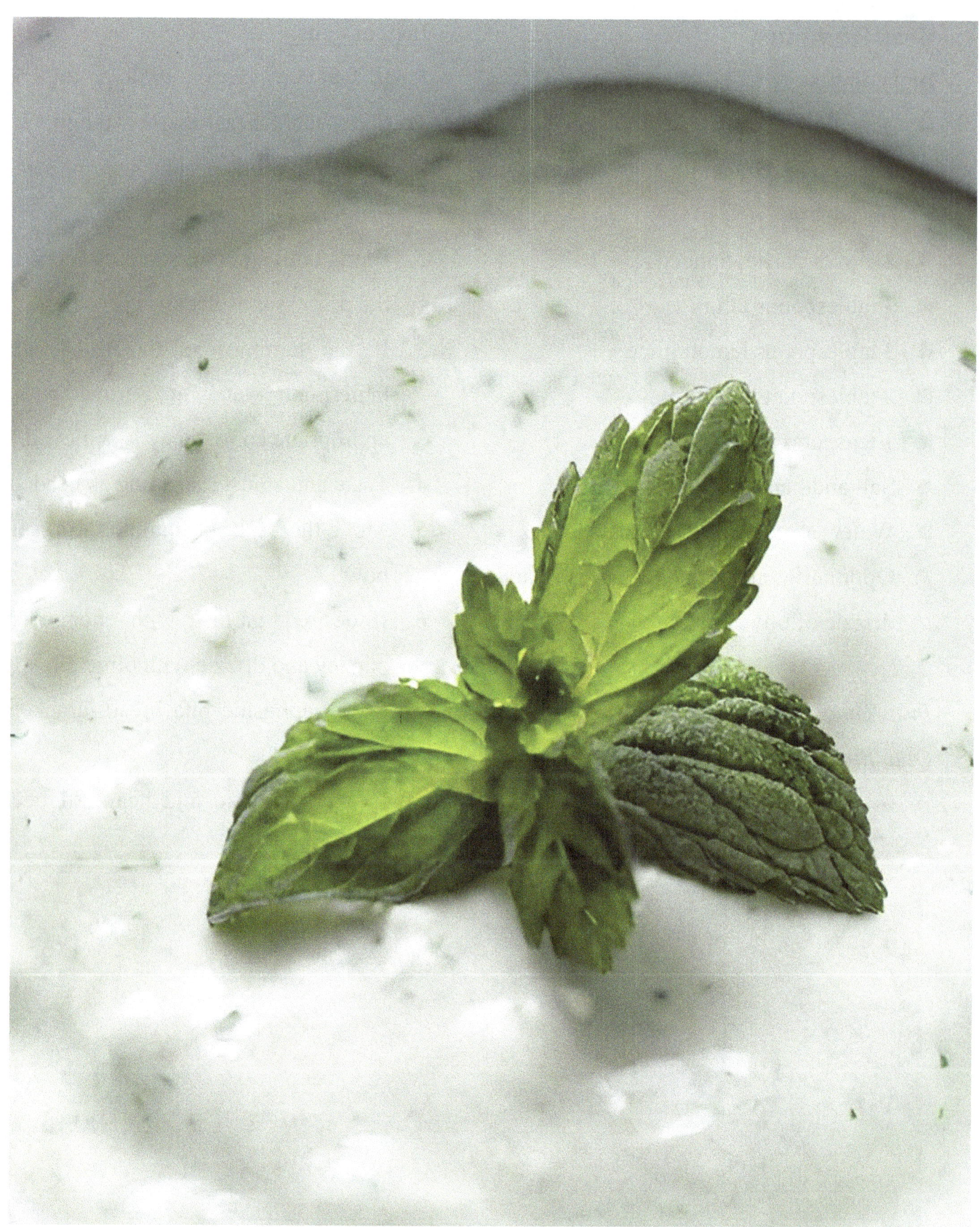

MEAT MAINS

Salmon with Walnut Crust:

Ingredients:

- 4 salmon fillets (about 6 ounces each)
- 1 cup chopped walnuts
- 1/4 cup grated Parmesan cheese
- 2 tablespoons chopped fresh parsley
- 1 tablespoon olive oil
- 1 tablespoon Dijon mustard
- Salt and pepper to taste
- Lemon wedges for serving

Prep Time: 10 minutes

Cook Time: 15 minutes

Total Time: 25 minutes

Servings: 4

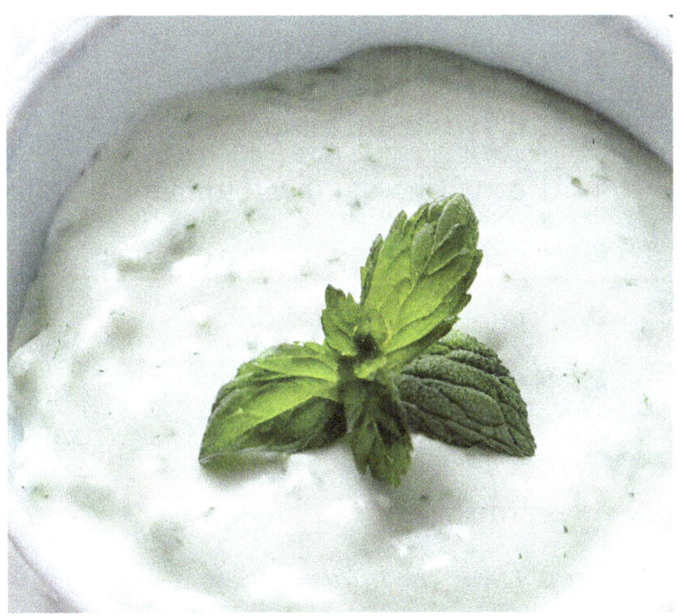

Instructions:

1. Preheat the oven to 400 °F (200 °C). Cover a baking sheet with parchment paper or lightly oil it.
2. In a bowl, combine the chopped walnuts, grated Parmesan cheese, chopped parsley, olive oil, Dijon mustard, salt, and pepper.
3. Place the salmon fillets on the prepared baking sheet.
4. Spread the walnut mixture evenly on top of each salmon fillet, gently pressing to adhere.
5. Bake for 12-15 minutes in a preheated oven, or until the salmon is fully cooked and the crust is golden brown.
6. Serve the salmon hot, with lemon wedges on the side to squeeze over the top.
7. Enjoy this tasty and healthful salmon with walnut crust!

Grilled Chicken with Spinach and Garlic:

Ingredients:

- 4 boneless, skinless chicken breasts
- 2 cups fresh spinach leaves
- 4 cloves garlic, minced
- 2 tablespoons olive oil
- Salt and pepper to taste

Prep time: 10 minutes

Cook time: 15 minutes

Total time: 25 minutes

Servings: 4

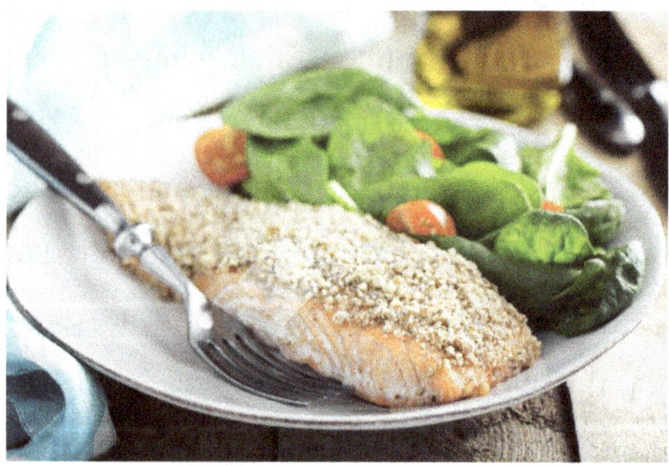

Instructions:

1. Preheat the grill to medium-high heat.
2. In a small bowl, combine the minced garlic and olive oil.
3. Season the chicken breasts with salt and pepper on both sides.
4. Brush garlic-infused olive oil on each chicken breast.
5. Grill the chicken for about 6-7 minutes per side, or until it is fully cooked and the juices run clear.
6. While the chicken grills, softly sauté the spinach in a pan until wilted.
7. Serve grilled chicken breasts hot, with sautéed spinach on the side.
8. Enjoy the tasty grilled chicken with spinach and garlic!

Turkey and Quinoa Stuffed Peppers:

Ingredients:

- 4 large bell peppers (any color)
- 1 pound ground turkey
- 1 cup cooked quinoa
- 1 onion, diced
- 2 cloves garlic, minced
- 1 can (14.5 oz) diced tomatoes, drained
- 1 cup shredded mozzarella cheese
- 1 tablespoon olive oil
- Salt and pepper to taste
- Optional: chopped fresh parsley for garnish

Prep Time: 15 minutes

Cook Time: 35 minutes

Total Time: 50 minutes

Servings: 4

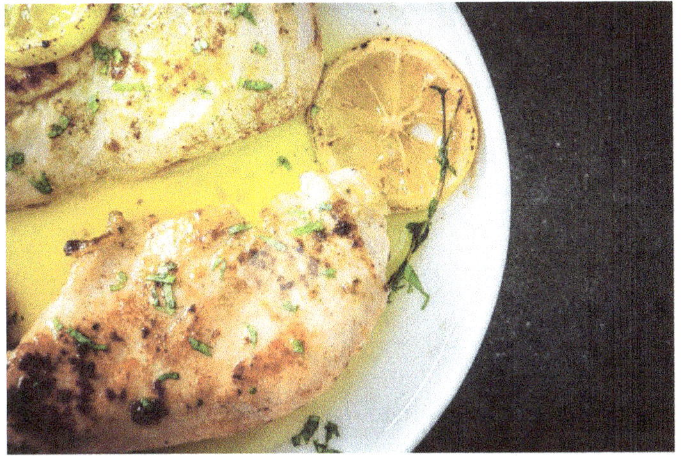

Instructions:

1. Preheat the oven to 375°F (190° C).

2. Cut the bell pepper tops off and remove the seeds and membranes. Put the peppers in a baking tray and set aside.

3. In a skillet, heat the olive oil over medium heat. Sauté sliced onion and minced garlic until tender.

4. Add the ground turkey to the skillet and heat until browned, breaking it up with a spoon as you go.

5. Stir in the cooked quinoa and diced tomatoes. Season with salt and pepper to taste. Cook for a another 2-3 minutes, until well heated.

6. Spoon the turkey and quinoa mixture into each bell pepper until they are completely full.

7. Sprinkle shredded mozzarella cheese on top of each filled pepper.

8. Cover the baking dish with aluminium foil and bake in the preheated oven for 25 minutes.

9. Remove the foil and bake for another 10 minutes, or until the cheese is melted and bubbling and the peppers are soft.

10. Garnish with chopped fresh parsley before serving. Enjoy your Turkey and Quinoa Stuffed Peppers.

Beef Stir-Fry with Broccoli and Cashews:

Ingredients:

- 1 lb (450g) beef steak, thinly sliced
- 2 cups broccoli florets
- 1/2 cup cashews
- 3 cloves garlic, minced
- 2 tablespoons soy sauce
- 1 tablespoon oyster sauce
- 1 tablespoon sesame oil
- 1 tablespoon cornstarch
- 2 tablespoons vegetable oil

- Salt and pepper, to taste
- Cooked rice, for serving

Prep Time: 15 minutes

Cook Time: 15 minutes

Total Time: 30 minutes

Servings: 4

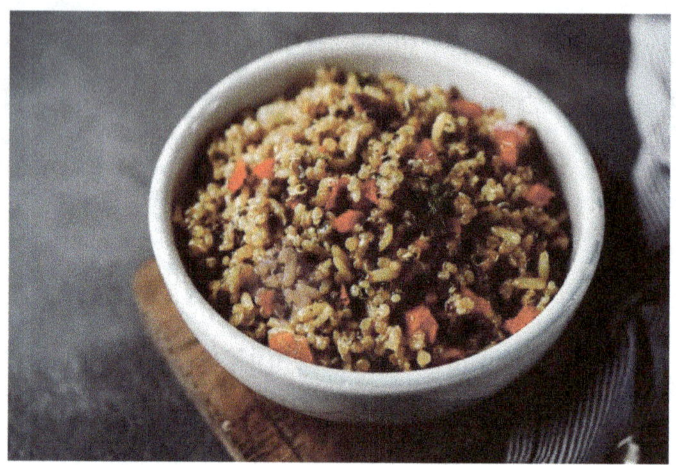

Instructions:

1. In a mixing bowl, add soy sauce, oyster sauce, sesame oil, minced garlic, and cornflour. Add the thinly sliced beef to the marinade, stir well, and leave aside for 10 minutes.

2. In a large skillet or wok, heat the vegetable oil on medium-high. Stir in the marinated beef and cook for 2-3 minutes, or until browned. Remove the steak from the skillet and put aside.

3. In the same skillet, cook broccoli florets for 2-3 minutes, until slightly cooked but still crisp.

4. Return the steak to the skillet alongside the broccoli. Add the cashews and whisk to mix.

5. Cook for an additional 2-3 minutes, or until everything is well cooked and coated with sauce.

6. Season with salt and pepper to taste.

7. Serve hot with prepared rice.

8. Enjoy this tasty beef stir-fry with broccoli and cashews!

Lemon Garlic Shrimp Skewers:

Ingredients:

- 1 lb large shrimp, peeled and deveined
- 3 cloves garlic, minced
- 2 tablespoons olive oil
- 2 tablespoons fresh lemon juice
- 1 teaspoon lemon zest
- Salt and pepper to taste
- Wooden skewers, soaked in water for 30 minutes

Prep Time: 15 minutes

Quantity: Makes 4 servings

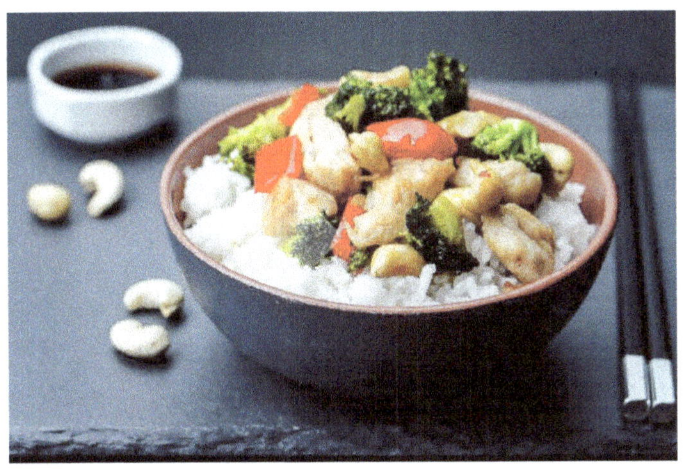

Instructions:

1. In a bowl, combine the minced garlic, olive oil, lemon juice, lemon zest, salt, and pepper.

2. Thread the prawns onto moistened wooden skewers, piercing both the tail and body.

3. Brush the garlic lemon mixture on the prawn skewers, making sure they are uniformly coated.

4. Preheat the grill to medium-high heat.

5. Grill prawn skewers for 2-3 minutes per side, or until they are pink and opaque.

6. Serve hot, topped with more lemon slices if preferred. Enjoy your lemon garlic prawn skewers!

Baked Turkey Meatballs with Tomato Sauce:

Ingredients:

- 1 lb ground turkey
- 1/2 cup breadcrumbs
- 1/4 cup grated Parmesan cheese
- 1 egg
- 2 cloves garlic, minced
- 1/4 cup chopped fresh parsley
- Salt and pepper to taste
- 1 tablespoon olive oil
- 1 can (15 oz) tomato sauce
- 1 teaspoon dried oregano
- 1/2 teaspoon dried basil
- Optional: grated mozzarella cheese for topping

Prep Time: 15 minutes

Quantity: Makes about 20 meatballs

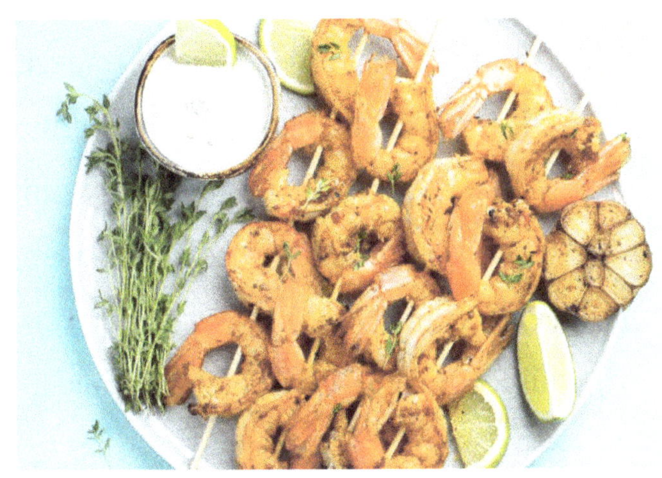

<u>**Instructions:**</u>

1. Preheat the oven to 375°F (190° C). Lightly grease or line a baking sheet with parchment paper.

2. In a large mixing bowl, combine ground turkey, breadcrumbs, Parmesan cheese, egg, minced garlic, chopped parsley, salt, and pepper. Mix thoroughly until all components are uniformly distributed.

3. Shape the mixture into meatballs that are 1 to 1.5 inches in diameter and set them on the prepared baking sheet.

4. In a separate bowl, combine the tomato sauce, dry oregano, and dried basil.

5. Spoon a little tomato sauce over each meatball, making sure it's equally coated.

6. Bake in the preheated oven for 20-25 minutes, or until the meatballs are thoroughly cooked.

7. If preferred, add grated mozzarella cheese over the meatballs during the last 5 minutes of baking for a cheesy finish.

8. Once done, remove from the oven and serve hot. Enjoy your tasty cooked turkey meatballs with tomato sauce!

Lamb Kebabs with Greek Salad:

<u>Ingredients:</u>

- 1 lb lamb, cut into cubes
- 1 red onion, cut into chunks
- 1 bell pepper, cut into chunks
- 1 zucchini, sliced
- 1/4 cup olive oil
- 2 tablespoons lemon juice
- 2 cloves garlic, minced
- 1 teaspoon dried oregano
- Salt and pepper to taste
- Wooden skewers, soaked in water

For Greek Salad:

- 2 large tomatoes, chopped
- 1 cucumber, diced
- 1/2 red onion, thinly sliced
- 1/2 cup Kalamata olives, pitted
- 1/2 cup crumbled feta cheese
- 2 tablespoons olive oil
- 1 tablespoon red wine vinegar
- 1 teaspoon dried oregano
- Salt and pepper to taste

Prep Time: 20 minutes

Quantity: 4 servings

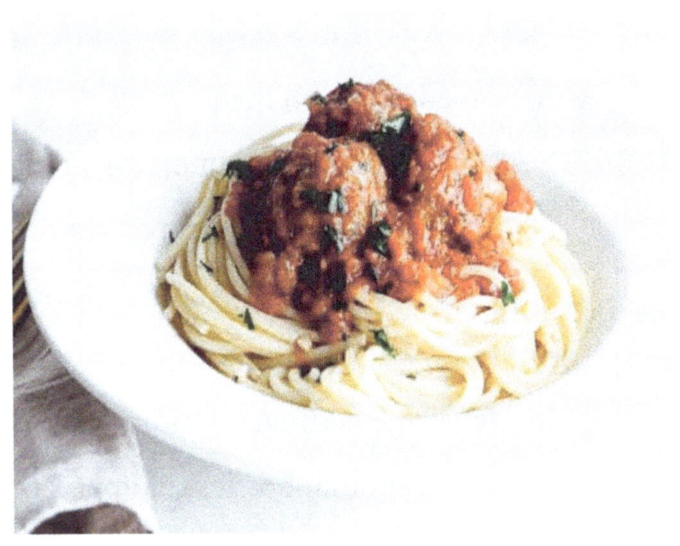

Instructions:

1. In a mixing bowl, combine olive oil, lemon juice, minced garlic, dried oregano, salt, and pepper. To create the marinade, thoroughly combine all ingredients.

2. Place the lamb cubes in a separate bowl and pour the marinade over them. Coat the lamb evenly. Allow to marinate for at least 30 minutes in the refrigerator.

3. Preheat the grill for medium-high heat.

4. Thread marinated lamb, red onion, red pepper and zucchini on moistened wooden skewers.

5. Grill the kebabs for 8-10 minutes, rotating regularly, until the lamb is cooked to your liking and the veggies are soft.

6. While the kebabs cook, make the Greek salad. In a large mixing bowl, combine chopped tomatoes, diced cucumber, thinly sliced red onion, Kalamata olives, and crumbled feta cheese.

7. To prepare the dressing, combine olive oil, red wine vinegar, dried oregano, salt, and pepper in a small bowl.

8. Pour the dressing over the salad and toss to mix.

9. Serve the grilled lamb kebabs with Greek salad on the side. Enjoy!

Pork Tenderloin with Apple Cranberry Chutney:

Ingredients:

- 1 pork tenderloin (about 1 to 1.5 lbs)
- 2 tablespoons olive oil
- Salt and pepper to taste

- 1 cup diced apples (peeled and cored)
- 1/2 cup dried cranberries
- 1/4 cup finely chopped onion
- 1/4 cup apple cider vinegar
- 2 tablespoons brown sugar
- 1/2 teaspoon ground cinnamon
- 1/4 teaspoon ground ginger

Prep Time: 10 minutes

Cook Time: 25 minutes

Total Time: 35 minutes

Servings: 4

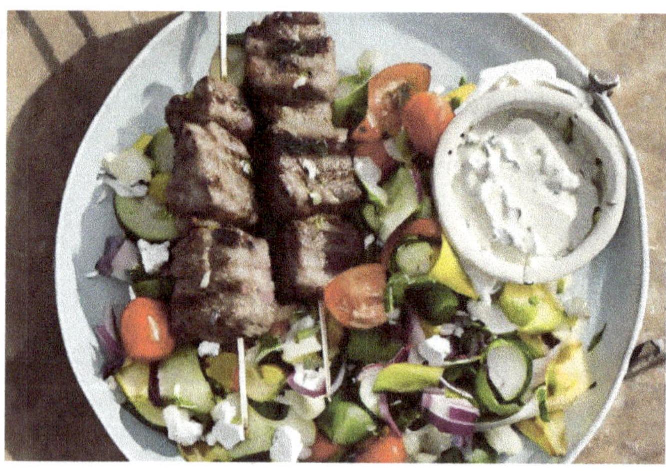

Instructions:

1. Preheat the oven to 400 °F (200 °C).
2. Season the pork tenderloin with salt and pepper.
3. Heat olive oil in a large oven-safe skillet over medium-high heat.
4. Sear the pork tenderloin on all sides until brown, about 2-3 minutes per side.
5. Remove the meat from the skillet and put aside.
6. In the same skillet, combine the diced apples, dried cranberries, chopped onion, apple cider vinegar, brown sugar, cinnamon, and ginger. Stir thoroughly.
7. Return the pork tenderloin to the skillet and nestle it in the apple cranberry mixture.
8. Place the skillet in the preheated oven and roast for 20-25 minutes, or until the pork registers an internal temperature of 145°F (63°C).
9. Remove the pan from the oven and allow the pork to rest for a few minutes before cutting.
10. Serve the sliced pork tenderloin with apple cranberry chutney spooned on top. Enjoy your great supper!

FISH AND SEAFOOD

Salmon Salad with Blueberries and Walnuts:

Ingredients:

- 2 salmon fillets
- 2 cups mixed greens
- 1/2 cup blueberries
- 1/4 cup chopped walnuts
- 1 tablespoon olive oil
- 1 tablespoon lemon juice
- Salt and pepper to taste

Prep Time: 15 minutes

Quantity: Serves 2

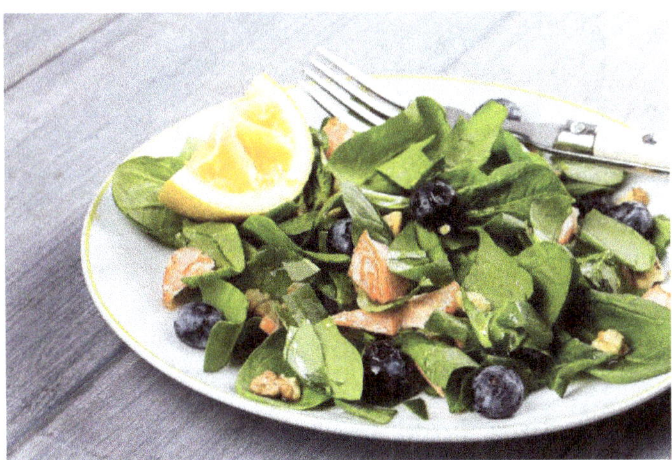

Instructions:

1. Preheat the oven to 400° F (200° C). Arrange the salmon fillets on a baking pan lined with parchment paper.

2. Drizzle the salmon with olive oil and lemon juice. Season with salt and pepper.

3. Bake the salmon for 12-15 minutes, or until thoroughly done.

4. In a large mixing basin, combine the greens, blueberries, and walnuts.

5. Once cooked, flake the salmon into bite-sized pieces and combine with the salad.

6. Drizzle with more olive oil and lemon juice if preferred. Toss gently until combined.

7. Serve immediately and enjoy your cool salmon salad with blueberries and walnuts.

Sardine and Avocado Toast:

Ingredients:

- 4 slices of whole grain bread
- 1 ripe avocado
- 1 can of sardines in olive oil
- Salt and pepper to taste
- Optional toppings: lemon juice, red pepper flakes, chopped parsley

Prep Time: 10 minutes

Quantity: Makes 4 slices of toast

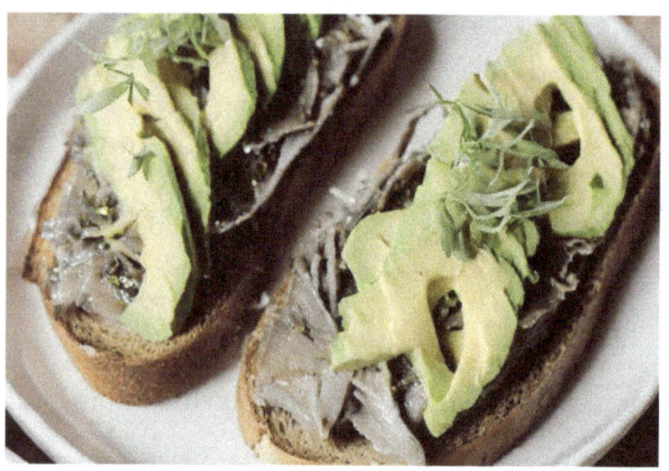

Instructions:

1. Toast whole grain bread until golden brown. Mash ripe avocado in a bowl with a fork.

2. Drain sardines from olive oil and remove any bones. After toasting, spread a generous layer of mashed avocado on each slice.

3. Top with sardines, dividing them evenly among the slices. Season with salt and pepper to taste.

4. Optional: Squeeze a bit of lemon juice.

Tuna and White Bean Salad:

Ingredients:

- 2 cans of tuna, drained
- 2 cans of white beans, drained and rinsed
- 1 red bell pepper, diced
- 1/4 cup red onion, finely chopped
- 1/4 cup fresh parsley, chopped
- 2 tablespoons lemon juice
- 2 tablespoons olive oil
- Salt and pepper to taste

Prep Time: 10 minutes

Quantity: Serves 4

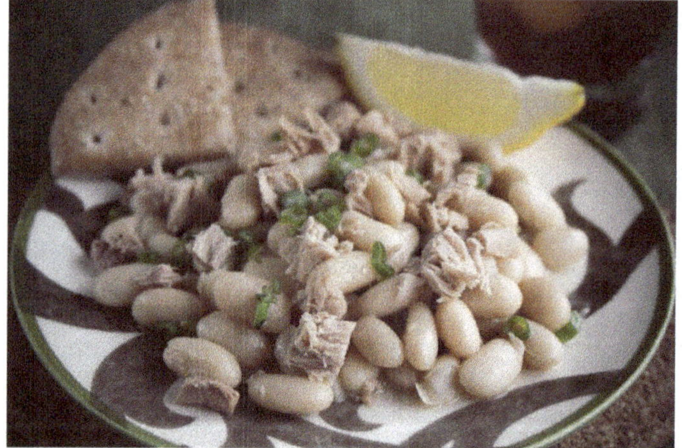

Instructions:

1. In a large mixing bowl, combine tuna, white beans, diced bell pepper, chopped red onion, and fresh parsley.

2. Drizzle lemon juice and olive oil over the mixture.

3. Season with salt and pepper to taste.

4. Gently toss all of the ingredients until completely combined.

5. Serve immediately or refrigerate until later. Enjoy!

Grilled Shrimp and Vegetable Skewers:

Ingredients:

- 1 pound large shrimp, peeled and deveined
- 2 bell peppers, assorted colors, cut into chunks
- 1 zucchini, sliced into rounds
- 1 red onion, cut into chunks
- 8-10 wooden skewers, soaked in water

For marinade:

- 1/4 cup olive oil
- 2 cloves garlic, minced
- 2 tablespoons lemon juice
- 1 teaspoon paprika
- Salt and pepper to taste
- Optional: chopped fresh herbs like parsley or cilantro for garnish

Prep Time: 15 minutes

Cook Time: 10 minutes

Total Time: 25 minutes

Servings: 4

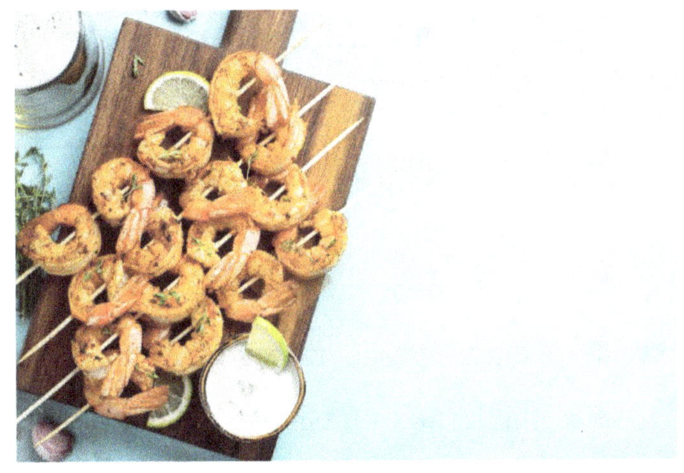

Instructions:

1. To make the marinade, combine olive oil, minced garlic, lemon juice, paprika, salt and pepper in a small bowl.

2. Thread shrimp, red peppers, zucchini slices and red onion chunks onto soaked wooden skewers, alternating between ingredients.

3. Place the assembled skewers in a shallow dish and pour the marinade over them, making sure they are well coated.

4. Allow to marinate for 10-15 minutes. Preheat grill to medium-high heat and grease the grill grate.

Baked Cod with Lemon and Herbs:

Ingredients:

- 4 cod fillets
- 2 lemons
- 2 tablespoons olive oil
- 2 cloves garlic, minced
- 1 tablespoon fresh parsley, chopped
- 1 tablespoon fresh dill, chopped
- Salt and pepper to taste

Prep Time: 10 minutes

Quantity: Serves 4

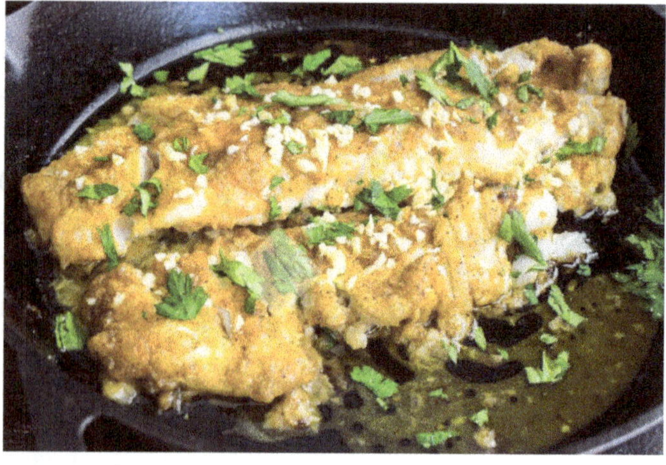

Instructions:

1. Preheat the oven to 375°F (190° C).
2. Put the cod fillets on a roasting tray.
3. Drizzle olive oil over the cod fillets.
4. Squeeze the juice of one lemon over each fillet.
5. Sprinkle the fillets evenly with minced garlic, chopped parsley, and chopped dill.
6. Season with salt and pepper to taste.
7. Thinly slice the second lemon and set it on top of the fillets.
8. Bake in the preheated oven for 15-20 minutes, or until the fish is cooked through and readily flaked with a fork.
9. Serve hot, topped with more lemon slices if preferred. Enjoy your tasty roasted cod with lemon and herbs!

Mackerel and Beetroot Salad:

Ingredients:

- 2 medium-sized cooked mackerel fillets, flaked
- 2 medium-sized cooked beetroots, sliced
- 2 cups mixed salad greens (such as arugula, spinach, or lettuce)
- 1/4 cup crumbled feta cheese
- 1/4 cup walnuts, chopped
- 2 tablespoons extra virgin olive oil
- 1 tablespoon balsamic vinegar
- Salt and pepper to taste

Prep Time: 15 minutes

Quantity: Serves 2

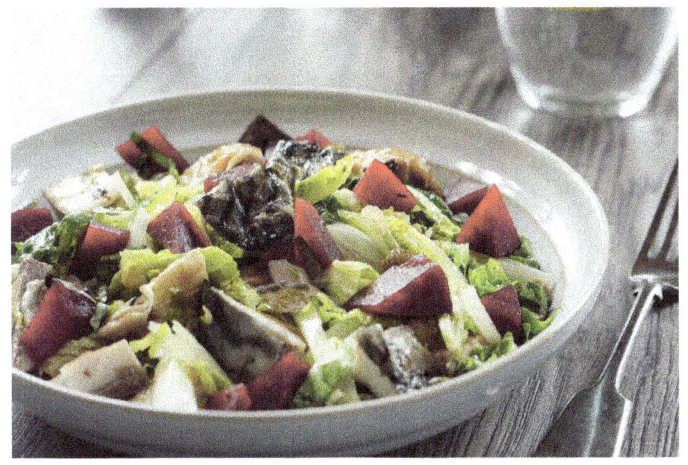

Instructions:

1. In a large mixing bowl, add the salad greens, sliced beetroots, and flakes mackerel.

2. Drizzle olive oil and balsamic vinegar over the salad.

3. Toss the salad gently to ensure that everything is coated equally.

4. Sprinkle the salad with crumbled feta cheese and chopped walnuts.

5. Season with salt and pepper to taste.

6. Serve immediately and enjoy your delicious Mackerel and Beetroot Salad.

Tilapia Tacos with Mango Salsa:

Ingredients:

- 4 tilapia fillets
- 8 small tortillas
- 1 ripe mango, diced
- 1/2 red onion, finely chopped
- 1/2 red bell pepper, diced
- 1/4 cup chopped fresh cilantro
- 1 jalapeño, seeded and minced
- Juice of 2 limes
- 1 tablespoon olive oil
- 1 teaspoon ground cumin
- Salt and pepper to taste

Prep Time: 20 minutes

Quantity: Makes 4 servings

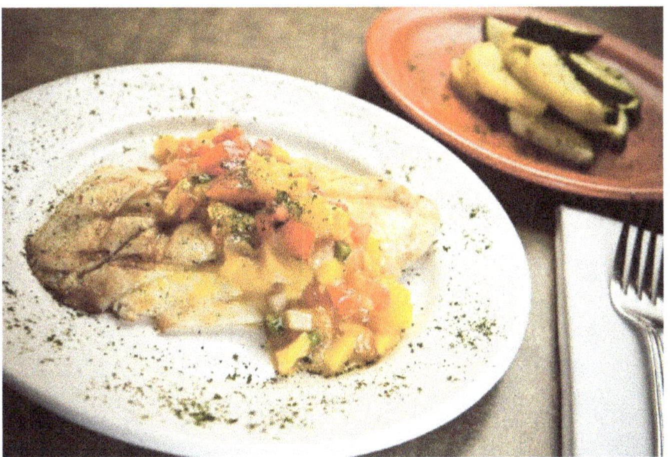

Instructions:

1. Preheat the grill or grill pan to medium-high heat.

2. To prepare mango salsa, combine chopped mango, red onion, red bell pepper, cilantro, jalapeño, and lime juice. Season with salt and pepper to taste.

3. Season tilapia fillets with olive oil, ground cumin, salt, and pepper.

4. Grill the tilapia fillets for 3-4 minutes per side, until they are cooked through and readily flaked with a fork.

5. Grill the tortillas for approximately 30 seconds on each side.

6. To make the tacos, lay one grilled tilapia fillet on each tortilla and top with mango salsa.

7. Serve immediately and enjoy your wonderful tilapia tacos with mango salsa.

Grilled Swordfish with Herb Pesto:

Ingredients:

- 4 swordfish fillets
- 2 tablespoons olive oil
- Salt and pepper to taste
- Lemon wedges for serving

For Herb Pesto:

- 2 cups fresh basil leaves
- 1/4 cup pine nuts
- 2 cloves garlic
- 1/2 cup grated Parmesan cheese
- 1/2 cup extra virgin olive oil
- Salt and pepper to taste

Prep Time: 15 minutes

Cook Time: 10 minutes

Total Time: 25 minutes

Servings: 4

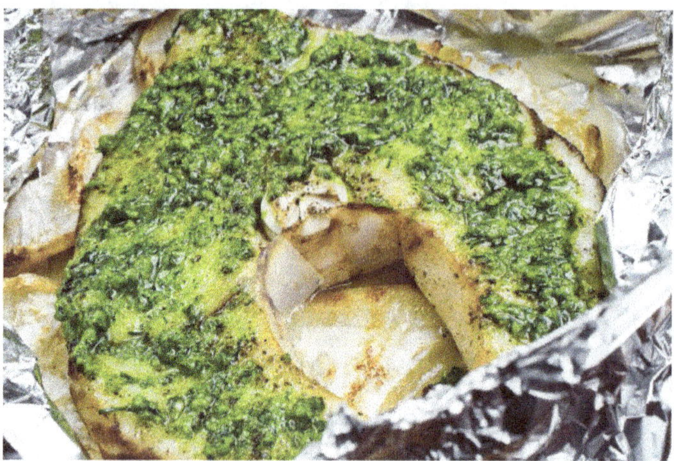

Instructions:

1. Preheat the grill to medium-high heat.

2. Season swordfish fillets with olive oil, salt, and pepper.

3. Grill the swordfish fillets for 4-5 minutes on each side, or until they are fully cooked and have grill marks.

4. While the swordfish grills, make the herb pesto. In a food processor, combine the basil leaves, pine nuts, garlic, Parmesan cheese, salt, and pepper. Pulse until finely chopped.

5. With the food processor running, slowly sprinkle in the olive oil until the pesto is smooth.

6. Once done, remove the swordfish from the grill and place on a serving plate.

7. Spread the herb pesto on the cooked swordfish fillets.

8. Serve immediately, with lemon slices to the side. Enjoy your Grilled Swordfish with Herbal Pesto!

Smoked Trout and Spinach Frittata:

Ingredients:

- 6 large eggs
- 1 cup smoked trout, flaked
- 1 cup fresh spinach, chopped
- 1/2 cup shredded cheddar cheese
- 1/4 cup milk
- 1 tablespoon olive oil
- Salt and pepper to taste

Prep Time: 10 minutes

Quantity: 4 servings

Instructions:

1. Preheat the oven grill.

2. In a mixing bowl, combine eggs, milk, salt, and pepper.

3. Heat the olive oil in an oven-safe skillet over medium heat.

4. Cook the spinach in the skillet for about 2 minutes, or until it has wilted.

5. Pour the egg mixture into a skillet.

6. Sprinkle the flakes trout and grated cheese equally over the eggs.

7. Cook until the edges begin to firm, about 3-4 minutes.

8. Place the skillet in the preheated oven and broil for 3-4 minutes, or until brown and the eggs are set.

9. Remove from the oven, let cool for a minute before slicing and serving hot. Enjoy your smoked trout and spinach frittata!

BONUS WEEK 4 MEAL PLAN

Focused on Promoting a Healthy Brain and Mind

WEEK 1	BREAKFAST	LUNCH	DINNER	SNACKS
Monday	Greek Yogurt with Berries	Grilled Salmon Salad	Quinoa Stir-fry with Veggies	Mixed Nuts
Tuesday	Oatmeal with Almond Butter	Turkey Wrap with Avocado	Baked Chicken with Sweet Potatoes	Carrot Sticks with Hummus
Wednesday	Spinach and Mushroom Omelette	Quinoa Salad with Chickpeas	Lentil Soup with Whole Grain Bread	Greek Yogurt with Honey
Thursday	Whole Grain Toast with Avocado	Grilled Chicken Quinoa Bowl	Broiled Fish with Steamed Broccoli	Apple Slices with Peanut Butter
Friday	Smoothie with Spinach, Banana, and Almond Milk	Veggie Stir-fry with Brown Rice	Stuffed Bell Peppers with Lean Ground Turkey	Trail Mix

WEEK 2	BREAKFAST	LUNCH	DINNER	SNACKS
Monday	Scrambled Eggs with Spinach	Quinoa and Black Bean Salad	Grilled Shrimp with Quinoa	Celery Sticks with Almond Butter
Tuesday	Whole Grain Pancakes with Berries	Chicken Caesar Salad	Baked Salmon with Asparagus	Greek Yogurt with Granola
Wednesday	Overnight Oats with Chia Seeds	Lentil Soup with Whole Grain Bread	Turkey Meatballs with Zucchini Noodles	Mixed Berries
Thursday	Breakfast Burrito with Beans and Veggies	Tuna Salad Wrap	Stir-fried Tofu with Vegetables	Cottage Cheese with Pineapple
Friday	Smoothie with Kale, Mango, and Greek Yogurt	Quinoa and Chickpea Stuffed Bell Peppers	Grilled Chicken with Sweet Potato Mash	Almonds

WEEK 3	BREAKFAST	LUNCH	DINNER	SNACKS
Monday	Acai Bowl with Fresh Fruit	Grilled Vegetable Wrap	Baked Cod with Quinoa Salad	Hard-boiled Eggs
Tuesday	Whole Grain Toast with Ricotta and Honey	Mediterranean Salad	Stir-fried Beef with Broccoli	Cottage Cheese with Berries
Wednesday	Spinach and Feta Frittata	Lentil Soup with Whole Grain Bread	Turkey Chili with Brown Rice	Apple Slices with Almond Butter
Thursday	Smoothie with Blueberries, Spinach, and Almond Milk	Chicken and Quinoa Bowl	Baked Chicken with Roasted Vegetables	Carrot Sticks with Hummus
Friday	Chia Seed Pudding with Fresh Berries	Greek Salad with Grilled Chicken	Stuffed Portobello Mushrooms	Trail Mix

WEEK 4	BREAKFAST	LUNCH	DINNER	SNACKS
Monday	Whole Grain Waffles with Peanut Butter	Quinoa Salad with Roasted Vegetables	Grilled Steak with Sweet Potato Fries	Greek Yogurt with Mixed Nuts
Tuesday	Avocado Toast with Poached Egg	Chicken Caesar Wrap	Baked Salmon with Quinoa	Apple Slices with Peanut Butter
Wednesday	Veggie Omelette with Whole Grain Toast	Lentil Soup with Whole Grain Bread	Turkey Stir-fry with Brown Rice	Cottage Cheese with Pineapple
Thursday	Smoothie with Banana, Spinach, and Almond Milk	Greek Salad with Grilled Shrimp	Baked Chicken with Steamed Vegetables	Mixed Berries
Friday	Overnight Oats with Mixed Berries	Tuna Salad Sandwich	Quinoa Stuffed Bell Peppers	Almonds

This meal plan includes a variety of nutrient-rich foods known for their brain-boosting properties, such as fruits, vegetables, whole grains, lean proteins, and healthy fats. It also offers a balance of macro-nutrients and incorporates snacks to keep energy levels stable throughout the day. Remember to adjust portion sizes and specific food choices based on individual dietary needs and preferences. Additionally, staying hydrated by drinking plenty of water throughout the day is essential for optimal brain function.

Blank Diet Meal Plan

CONCLUSION

Embracing the Mind Diet Lifestyle

Incorporating Mindful Eating Habits

Mindful eating entails developing a greater awareness of your eating habits, sensations, and the relationship between food and your body. Mindfulness during meals can improve your general well-being, digestion, and foster a healthier connection with food. Here's a complete guide on incorporating mindful eating practices into your lifestyle:

Begin with Awareness: Become more conscious of your eating behaviours, including when, when, why, and what you consume. Observe any patterns or triggers that influence your food choices and eating habits.

Eat Slowly: Slow down your eating pace to properly savour and appreciate each bite. Chew your meal thoroughly, focusing on the flavours, textures, and sensations in your mouth.

Reduce Distractions: Avoid using television, smartphones, or other electronic devices during meals. Concentrate exclusively on the process of eating and the sensation of fueling your body.

Engage Your Senses: To truly savour your cuisine, use all of your senses. Consider the colours, smells, and sounds of your meal. Engaging your senses can increase your enjoyment and contentment with food.

Practice thankfulness: Before you start eating, take a moment to express your thankfulness for the food in front of you. Consider the labour that went into creating and preparing your food, and appreciate the nutrition it delivers to your body.

Listen to your body's hunger and fullness cues. Eat when you're hungry and stop when you're full, rather than waiting for external cues or eating everything on your plate out of habit.

Mindful Portion Control: Pay attention to portion sizes and offer yourself the appropriate amount of food. Use smaller dishes and utensils to regulate portion sizes and avoid overeating.

Mindful Snacking: Practice mindfulness during snacking by selecting healthful foods and eating them without interruptions. Consider how your body feels before, during, and after snacking, and then alter your habits accordingly.

Be Nonjudgmental: Practice self-compassion and avoid having judgmental thoughts or attitudes regarding your eating habits. Accept yourself and your decisions with respect and understanding, and concentrate on making positive adjustments going forward.

Cultivate Mindful Eating traditions: Create mealtime traditions, such as setting the table, lighting a candle, or saying a grace or affirmation before eating. These routines can send a signal to your brain that it's time to calm down and enjoy your food.

Mindful Eating Meditation: Add mindful eating to your meditation practice by taking a few minutes to consume a single piece of food thoughtfully. Take note of every sensation you feel while eating, from the moment the food enters your mouth until you swallow.

Practice Consistency: Mindful eating, like any other habit, requires practice and consistency to establish. Aim to include mindfulness into your meals on a daily basis, even if only for a few minutes at first, and progressively expand the duration over time.

Seek Help: Consider attending a mindful eating group or consulting with a dietitian or therapist who specializes in mindful eating. Surrounding yourself with support and guidance will help you maintain your mindful eating habits and stay encouraged on your path.

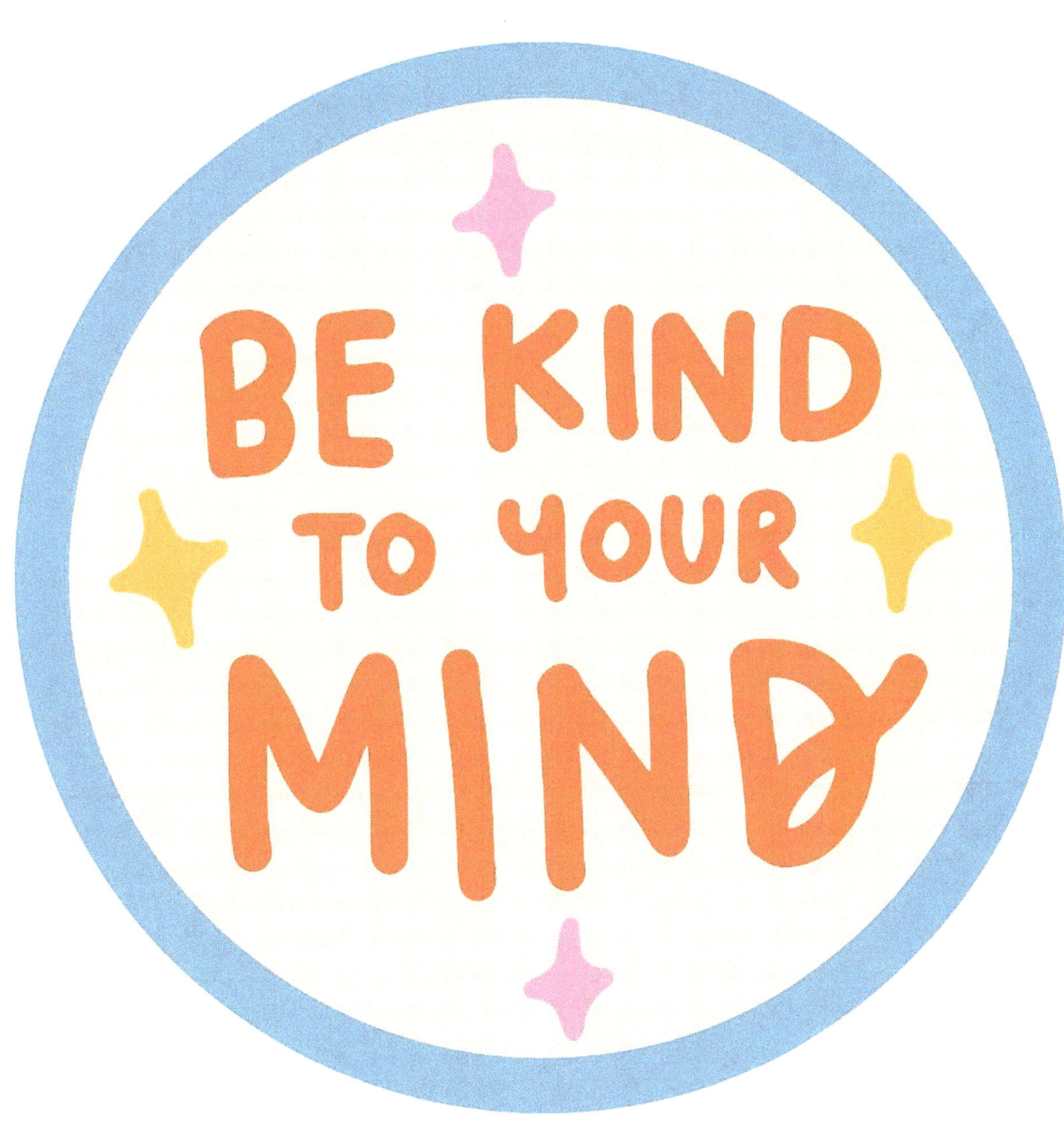